Machine readable labels in the blood transfusion service

Travenol Laboratories are pleased to have been associated with this symposium and the publication of its proceedings.

Beginning with the introduction of the Fenwall Blood System for the safe collection, processing and administration of blood and blood components, we are proud of the contribution we have made to the rapid progress seen in blood tranfusion practice and blood component therapy.

Our participation in the introduction of computer linked programmes to further improve identification and control of blood and blood components using a bar-code system will enable us to continue to develop the working relationship established with the NBTS and to jointly contribute to significant advances in transfusion practice.

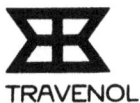

TRAVENOL

Machine readable labels in the blood transfusion service

Proceedings of a Symposium
held on June 13th, 1979

Edited by John Jenkins
Director North East Thames
Regional Transfusion Centre

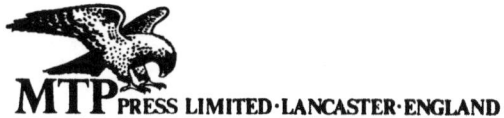

MTP PRESS LIMITED·LANCASTER·ENGLAND

Published by
MTP Press Limited
Falcon House
Lancaster, England

Copyright © 1980 MTP Press Limited

First Published 1980

British Library Cataloguing in Publication Data

Codabar Meeting, *Broadway, Worcs. 1979*
  Machine readable labels in the blood
  transfusion service.
  1. Blood banks — Great Britain — Congresses
  2. Machine readable labels — Congresses
  I. Title II. Jenkins, John
  615' 6507   RM172

ISBN 978-0-85200-344-2   ISBN 978-94-009-8046-4 (eBook)
DOI 10.1007/978-94-009-8046-4

Contents

INTRODUCTION
Dr W J Jenkins

In 1977 when the Sheffield Transfusion Centre took delivery of the first GROUPAMATIC blood grouping machine in the UK it was equipped with a sample identification system involving complicated and expensive disposable punched cards. In fact, the cards were so expensive that Dr Wagstaff was unable to find the revenue to support the system. A year later, when Brentwood took delivery of a GROUPAMATIC, we were faced with the same problem, but by chance we heard that KONTRON was developing a laser scanning system for bar code labels and we were able to have our machine modified. Subsequently the Sheffield machine was altered to take the bar code scanner.

At about the same time the Bristol Centre was helping TECHNICON with the development of the AUTO GROUPER C-16, and fortunately they decided on a laser reader of the same type for bar code identification. Thus there were three centres with the capability for reading bar codes on blood grouping machines and it became necessary to find someone to produce the bar code labels. There was only one printer in the UK who could produce labels to the required specification. To cut the costs of printing, and in the hope of avoiding a wide variation in codes, I invited representatives of centres interested in the problem to a meeting, where we set up what we called the Group of Six. This later became an official Working Party of the Regional Transfusion Directors.

The Working Party has been very active and has shown a degree of co-operation, the like of which I have never before witnessed in the NBTS. We realised that most of the hard work had already been done by our American colleagues, and we adopted the principles laid down by the CCBBA - The Committee for Commonality in Blood Bank Automation.

Today's meeting has been promoted with three objectives in mind. First, to provide an opportunity to hear the views of Dr Eric Brodheim, who was chairman of that American Committee, and to learn from his mistakes in applying the system in the New York Blood Centre.

The second objective was to allow members of our own Working Party to express their views to a wider audience within the NBTS and under more convivial circumstances than we might find at the Elephant and Castle. The third was to allow members of the Working Parties to receive the views of other centres and to incorporate new ideas as we go along.

Transfusion accidents still occur and those that occur today are most often due to organisational or transcription errors. The introduction of sample identification techniques in blood grouping machines, when linked with the use of light pens and microprocessors, can go a long way towards eliminating this hazard, and the system lends itself to full computerisation of blood bank inventory control.

The obvious way to start such a meeting is with an explanation of what bar coding is, and how it works. I therefore have pleasure in calling Mrs Jackson to talk about Technical Aspects of Bar Coding.

TECHNICAL ASPECTS OF BAR CODING

Mrs S Jackson (Regional Transfusion Centre, Birmingham)

Mrs JACKSON: I do not like the term 'expert'. There is an expert in the audience who knows far more about it than I do, ie Dr Brodheim. May I ask him to bail me out if I am putting across any information that is not strictly accurate.

I shall try to give some explanation of bar coding and some idea of the areas in which we apply bar coding in the blood transfusion centres.

As Dr Jenkins has already said, blood transfusion centres are in the business of collecting blood and supplying it to hospitals for eventual transfusion to patients. The great danger in this process is the possibility of transfusing a patient with incompatible blood. Transfusion centres, therefore, are geared to extensively analysing and identifying the individual characteristics of each unit of blood collected and to passing on this information to the hospitals. This information is conveyed by means of labels that are attached to each blood pack.

As has already been said, if errors are to occur, it is not so much in the laboratory processes where the actual analysis is made, but rather in the clerical processes where this information is read, or transcribed, and where labels are actually attached to the packs. These are the areas where errors occur, and these are the areas where we need to try to improve accuracy to increase our security.

The most effective way of achieving this would seem to be to introduce automated methods where possible when processing blood donations. This will involve the introduction of automatic blood grouping machines, and possibly the introduction of a computer to store and reproduce laboratory findings. The computer can also be used to control the issue and distribution of the eventual blood products that we produce.

Three items of information which are particularly critical have been identified as an aid to improving accuracy and security of information.

These are:

- the unique identification number which is allocated to each donation;
- the blood group and rhesus factor;
- the eventual blood product.

These three items ultimately appear on the blood packs which are sent out to the hospitals.

Take the donation identification number. Once this has been allocated to a donation, it is the link between the blood donor, the blood products, and the blood recipient, and it will be referred to many times during the course of processing. It is essential that each time the number is referred to, it is interpreted accurately. One way to ensure this is to make the number not only readable by the human eye but also readable by automated equipment, by blood grouping machines and by computers. The part of the number that the automated equipment reads is the part that is called the bar code. The same argument applies to blood group and to blood product. Once these have been determined and the blood pack has been labelled with this information, it is essential that the label is consistently and accurately interpreted, and it is for this reason that both blood group and blood product labels will also carry a machine-readable bar code.

Bar Coding

I have spoken of the need to improve accuracy and of the need for greater security. Coincidentally, by introducing bar coding, we have also introduced a fast method of capturing information. Bar codes can be read by automatic blood grouping machines by a laser scanner, and for the computer they can be read by light pen attachment. Both laser scanners and light pens pass a beam of light across the bar codes, and the information is instantaneously recorded in a digital form.

This is a much faster method of recording information than by manual transcription, and it is much faster than the more traditional method of capturing information for automated equipment where we would use a keyboard.

Finally, for those who have purchased, or are about to purchase, an automatic blood grouping machine, as has already been said, an integral part of the design of these machines is that they require blood samples to be labelled with bar-coded labels. Those who are planning to use automatic blood grouping machines are now in a position where they must use bar codes.

4

Let me attempt to give some definition of bar coding. A machine-readable linear bar code has printed lines and spaces arranged in different ways to represent different characters. These codes are read by laser scanner or light pen which are very sensitive to the variations in the light and the dark areas within the bar code.

Bar coding is not new. It has been around for some time now. Stock control systems use it in the retail trade. It is used at point of sale. Stores such as Comet and several of the larger supermarkets are looking at using bar codes, labelling items with bar codes and checking them out at the cashpoints. It has been used in libraries. It has been used for hospital patient identification. The Stoke-on-Trent project uses bar codes to identify patients there. It has also been used for laboratory sample identification.

There are many different types of bar code. When I first looked at bar codes the two which were probably fairly common in the UK were the Plessey bar code and a code called TELEPEN, marketed by SB Electronics. It was at about this time that we became aware of the work that was being done by the Committee for Commonality in Blood Bank Automation, or the CCBBA.

We have benefited a great deal from the work of this Committee. They started in January 1974 and they produced their final report in 1977. Those were three years of extensive work involving a lot of people and have proved extremely valuable to us. Their aims and objectives are exactly the same as ours. They want to improve the accuracy and the security of the products that they produce.

The CCBBA have not only reported on the introduction of bar codes, but they have also made recommendations for standard label designs and for standard numeric code allocations for blood groups and blood products, all of which we have been able to utilise.

With regard to the bar code, the CCBBA has set up a special Symbol Selection Task Force which investigated a number of different machine-readable symbols before recommending Codabar as the code most suitable for blood transfusion services. The criteria they used to evaluate the different codes that were available included ease of printing of the code. When we came to look at bar codes there was only one printer in the UK who could actually produce the labels. Ideally we should be able to use on-site printers to produce bar codes, rather than to have to keep going out to manufacturers.

They looked, too, at how easy the code was to use. Obviously it is no good labelling the blood pack with bar codes if, when one picks up a pen, one fails to get a read first time and must go through the code two or three times before getting the information transmitted. The Committee, therefore, set their sights at a 'first time read rate' in the region of 95-99 per cent as being an acceptable standard.

They looked at how accurately the light pen or the laser scanner could interpret the code. It is no good reading a bar code and then having the information wrongly transmitted.

They looked at the codes in the light of the blood transfusion service. Could the codes be used to record such things as donation numbers, blood groups, blood products? Was it a suitable structure of code for our uses.

Codabar was the code that measured up to the criteria most satisfactorily.

The details of the Committee's investigations and the details of the criteria that were set are to be found in the CCBBA Final Report, Volume 3.

Having selected Codabar, the Committee then modified the Code so that it met the requirements of blood transfusion services more exactly. The resultant code is known as the ABC (American Blood Commission) symbol.

The ABC symbol is a linear bar code which uses straight black vertical bars with white spaces to represent items of information. Each symbol is represented by four bars and three spaces, and these bars and spaces are either wide or narrow in dimension. Each set of seven wide and narrow bars and spaces represents one character.

Bar coding – why do we need it?

- Improved accuracy
- Greater security
- Speed
- Automatic blood grouping machines

Example of character set assignments

Number	7 Bar code	Bar pattern
1	0000110	
2	0001001	

When a narrow bar and a wide bar are compared, the wide bar is represented by a binary 1 and the narrow bar by a binary 0. Similarly with the spaces. A wide space has a binary 1 and a narrow space a binary 0. A 7-bit pattern of 0's and 1's represents each number.

The full ABC character symbol set includes twenty characters: Numeric 0 through 9, special characters such as colons, dollar signs, fullstops, etc, and a set of four characters, A, B, C and D which are referred to as start/ stop codes.

When an item of information is recorded, it must be preceded by a start code and it must be finished with a stop code. That is so that the light pen can recognise the start and the finish of any message.

These are called start/stop codes, because any message can be read in either directon. If a number is recorded the light pen has to be capable of reading it it from left to right or from right to left and still put over the information correctly.

Start and stop codes are not normally a part of the eye-readable message. Any bar code that is assigned will have an eye-readable interpretation along with it. Start and stop codes only appear in the bars. They do not appear in the eye-readable information under normal circumstances.

As an additional security measure, the ABC symbol has further modified the start and stop characters. Apparently it is possible, when a hand-held light pen is passed across a message, for the pen to wander out of the message and come back in again - and still give a valid read. The ABC symbol therefore recommends that these start and stop codes should be unique to each type of information, or to each type of message, and to achieve that it has proved necessary to allocate numeric control characters to be used in conjunction with the start and stop codes.

ABC Symbol – full character set

0-9	Zero through nine	**a**	Start or Stop code
:	Colon	**b**	Start or Stop code
+	Plus sign	**c**	Start or Stop code
$	Dollar sign	**d**	Start or Stop code
—	Minus sign		
.	Full stop		
/	Slash		

We are talking about recording donor identification numbers, blood groups, blood product codes, and centre identifications with bar codes.

The donor identification number has allocated to it a D-start and a D-stop code. Blood groups have D-starts and OB-stops. Blood products have AO-start and 2B-stops. The centre identification code has an AO-start and an 1B-stop. When the light pen reads a message, then if it reads, say, a D-start and a D-stop, it knows that the information it has picked up is a donor identification number and that it should be seven characters in length. Similarly with blood groups. If it recognises a D-start and a OB-stop, it knows that this is blood group code and should be two characters in length. Similarly with blood product codes. These should have five digits of information. The centre identification code should have seven digits.

The D-start and the D-stop have no accompanying control character, as with the Bs or the As. This is because the D-start and the D-stop characters have a special function, sometimes referred to as a pause code. This can be most clearly seen by considering the labelling of a blood pack with donor identification number and blood group code. When the two labels are attached to the pack, the donation identification number is placed adjacent to the blood group so that the bar codes are next to each other. When the light pen is passed across the two labels, it goes from the start of the donation identification number straight through to the stop code of the blood group code, and it transmits that information as one message.

The D-stop code on the donation identification number, and the D-start code at the beginning of the blood group are next to each other. The light pen must detect the D-start a fraction of a second after it has detected the D-stop. There is a reason for that. Once the identification number has been read, there should not be the time to lift the pen off the blood pack and on to somewhere else before it reads the blood group.

Control code assignments

d – 7 digit donation identification number   d

d	...	O	POS	(51)	...	Ob
d	...	A	POS	(62)	...	Ob
d	..,	B	POS	(73)	...	Ob
d	...	AB	POS	(84)	...	Ob
d	...	O	NEG	(95)	...	Ob
d	...	A	NEG	(06)	...	Ob
d	...	B	NEG	(17)	...	Ob
d	...	AB	NEG	(28)	...	Ob

aO – 5 digit blood product code   2b

aO – 7 digit transfusion centre identification number   1b

I hope I have explained what the start and the stop codes do, and that I have given some idea of the make-up of the information within a particular bar code.

Let me take each item of information independently. First, the security of each item. I have mentioned that the start and the stop codes provide some measure of security because they identify the type of information that was recorded. Because the donation identification number has a D-start and a D-stop it will be recognised as a donation identification number rather than a centre identification number, which has different start and stop codes, although both have seven digits. However, donation identification numbers are used frequently during the processing of any individual donation, and in many cases it will be necessary to record that information manually, particularly at hospital level where they may not be equipped to read the number with a light pen or a laser scanner. The problem with recording information by hand is that there is a possibility of transposition of numbers and of number substitution. The CCBBA therefore recommend that a check digit should be incorporated into that number.

There is apparently also a possibility, which is rated at 1 in 10^6, of the light pen being responsible for number substitution. It is estimated that the introduction of the check digit into the bar code will reduce this possibility to 1 in 10^9.

The advantages of using a check digit in conjunction with the donation identification number have to be weighed against the disadvantages of increasing that number to eight digits, which will create problems in handling the number, particularly at hospital level. As a group we have had a lot of discussion about the possibility of introducing check digits and the general feeling is that seven digits is already too many for handling at hospital level, and that it is not desirable to increase it to eight. To be honest, no satisfactory conclusion has yet been reached. In Birmingham they have elected not to include the check digit in the bar code because they are fairly happy that the light pen will transmit the information accurately, but the check digit has been included in the eye-readable message because they are not satisfied that when the number is being copied down manually the information will be accurately written accross. It is not yet resolved but it is a recommendation that in order to increase the security of that particular number, a check digit should be included.

The blood group code has the security of being identified by its own start and stop codes, and the number allocations for each blood group include additional security. Not only is that number unique, but if the numbers should be

9

transposed they would give numbers which are not valid blood group codes. No
transposition in those numbers will produce another valid code.

A lot of thought and a lot of care has been put into designing these codes in
order to ensure their security.

The blood product code, a five-digit code, is again unique because of its start
and stop characters. The actual format of the five digits is fairly complex.
The first three digits identify the product itself. The fourth digit identifies
either the anti-coagulant or the method of preparation. The fifth digit is used
to identify the package type or the volume. The actual breakdown and the way in
which the code is made up can be found in the CCBBA Report where it is fairly
extensively explained.

The blood transfusion centre identification code is distinguishable from the
other seven-digit number by its start and stop codes. It is made up of two digits
which identify the area of the UK in which the centre is situated: 70 for England,
 71 for Scotland, 72 for Northern Ireland, and 73 for Wales. The next two digits
identify the fourteen major transfusion centres by the use of the two-digit DHSS
number. The last three digits are available to identify sub-centres within
transfusion services where they exist.

These code allocations have been accepted by the six transfusion centres that
make up the Working Group and they are also in use in the USA, and there is now
in existence an international body that controls the use and the allocation of
these codes. If we need an extension to any of the coding structures, either for
additional blood groups, or blood products, or whatever, it will have to be
referred to this international committee which will allocate the number as
necessary and will control the make up of these codes.

I hope I have been able to convey some understanding of bar coding and some idea
of the way in which codes have been allocated to the various items of information
that we think it necessary to record. The make up of the codes and what I have
had to say about them should show that a lot of effort has been put into making
sure that this information is as accurate and as secure as it can possibly be.

PROPOSED CHANGES TO BLOOD PACK LABELS IN THE UK
Mrs A Wild (Travenol Laboratories)

Mrs WILD: Before I embark on my brief contribution to today's meeting, I must first introduce myself. I am Audrey Wild and I work with Scientific Services at Travenol, in Thetford, as Labelling Controller. As such I have been involved in the design and provision of blood pack labels compatible with the requirements of the Codabar Working Committee, and also along the lines of the recommendation of the CCBBA.

The new labelling is the result of teamwork between all the qualified members of the Labelling Group, but the final quality of the printed label can only be assured by discussions and co-operation between ourselves and our approved printers, especially where specific printing skills are involved, such as the provision of Codabar symbols.

I should like firstly to give you some idea of how we approached the Codabar project, and secondly, to introduce the new labels; as I call them - hybrid labels. These are labels which, with eye readable and machine readable information, can be properly used by all centres whether or not they are geared to automated blood banking systems. Finally, I shall look into the future, with the aim of achieving the ultimate simple label, providing uniformity but retaining the flexibility required by individual centres.

We are all obviously familiar with the overall objectives of eliminating the possibility of human error from before the drawing of blood up to the moment of transfusion, by the implementation of a Donor-blood Product-Recipient Identification System using simplified uniform labelling incorporating machine-readable symbols.

We, as suppliers of Fenwal blood packs, became involved in the project soon after the initiation of the Codabar Working Party, and our commitment was to redesign our traditional Fenwal labels so that they would still be acceptable to centres using conventional systems, and at the same time be equally acceptable to centres using conventional systems and those adopting the CCBBA approach to GROUPAMATIC units; this with the provision of both eye-readable and machine-readable information.

The new label was to be designed to provide the most efficient and logical placement of vital information with the correct emphasis on those statements of greatest importance. All product information at this stage, formulation of anti-coagulation, instructions, storage, and warnings were still to be retained on the label.

As our guide, we followed the CCBBA proposals, although these have been necessarily modified by the specific requirements of the centres involved. We have worked in very close co-operation with the Working Party at all times, and the labels which we are now presenting on our single, double and triple blood packs and their transfer packs have been the result of mutual agreements between all parties involved. Any changes, albeit minor, which have been made on textual content are still in strict conformance to British standards, DHSS specifications, and pharmacopoeial monographs.

In this, our first stage of the simplified label, the only preprinted Codabar symbol which we are implementing is the product code, such as CPD Whole Blood. This information is also clearly displayed in red eye-readable form. However, the Codabar symbol, in addition, also incorporates information defining the anti-coagulant and the blood pack unit type.

As the blood pack and its satellite packs progress through the blood processing system, the initial label becomes a basic matrix for the addition of hand-written or eye and machine readable overstick labels. The basic label and the design of the overstick labels must therefore be mutually compatible, and in order to preserve the integrity of our labels we are similarly concerned in ensuring the uniform design and integrity of the over labels. The positioning of the relevant Codabar symbols should, by the label design, allow the concurrent reading of information between two or more labels by a single pass of the light pen, and the controlled print quality of the symbol should ensure its readability. I do emphasise this point of the controlled print quality. This is difficult to achieve, but it is essential for the control of the system.

As one of the prime objectives of the CCBBA proposals is to reduce the possibility of error within the blood centres, it is our responsibility at Travenol as suppliers of blood packs to ensure the quality of our Codabar labels, and this we achieve by submitting each label to the highest possible control from its origination on the drawing board to the application of the label to the blood pack.

As has already been explained, the Codabar symbol was initially chosen because it was an extremely safe symbol which we aim will give a first pass read rate of 99 per cent per character. This read rate must be under all conditions to which blood packs are subjected during their normal use, and to ensure this we have examined all apsects of the new label, including choice of paper, the initiation and procurement of Codabar symbol masters, the establishing of printing techniques to ensure reproducability and readability of the symbol during successive production runs and control systems.

As far as the paper is concerned, initially this must show resistance to scratching and scuffing which would otherwise impair the readability of the symbol. Pasteurisation during the process of producing the blood packs and refrigeration at the centres both cause heavy condensation which precludes the use of a paper that might be porous. The hard glazed surface of the paper which we use at Travenol, and which is approved, minimizes any effect that the frequent rubbing of the light pen might cause, and after wetting, the label dries quickly, so that as the blood pack is taken from the refigerator, the integrity of the Codabar symbol should not be impaired.

The paper surface also has the added advantage of allowing symbols which have been over-labelled during the progress of the blood packs through the system to be destroyed in the event of the over labels being removed. This is essential to the integrity.

In addition, the design of the label had to be such that in areas where overstick labels with Codabar symbols would be placed, the readability of the uppermost symbol would not be threatened by underlying print showing through and invalidating the symbol.

Another point on this. When the label is applied to the blood bag, with blood, the dark colour of the blood must not impair the integrity of the symbol. The thickness of the paper and the opacity are critical.

To achieve this end, we worked in close co-operation with our printers to ensure that the symbols are controlled from initiation to print.

The Codabar symbols as specified initially by ourselves are electronically produced on film and supplied direct to the printer. These are positioned on art work drawn up by ourselves, by our own designer within our department, and from these negatives and plates are made. Before the printer is authorised to print, proofs must be scanned and verified, and approved by ourselves in the Labelling Group at Travenol, thereby establishing the control of the correctness of the symbols used. During printing, symbols are scanned on line during the actual runs by a Monarch Verifier unit, and statistical checks using a similar scanner are carried out in-house as part of routine Quality Control procedure. The integrity of the Codabar symbol is therefore controlled from its conception to its implementation on the labelled blood pack.

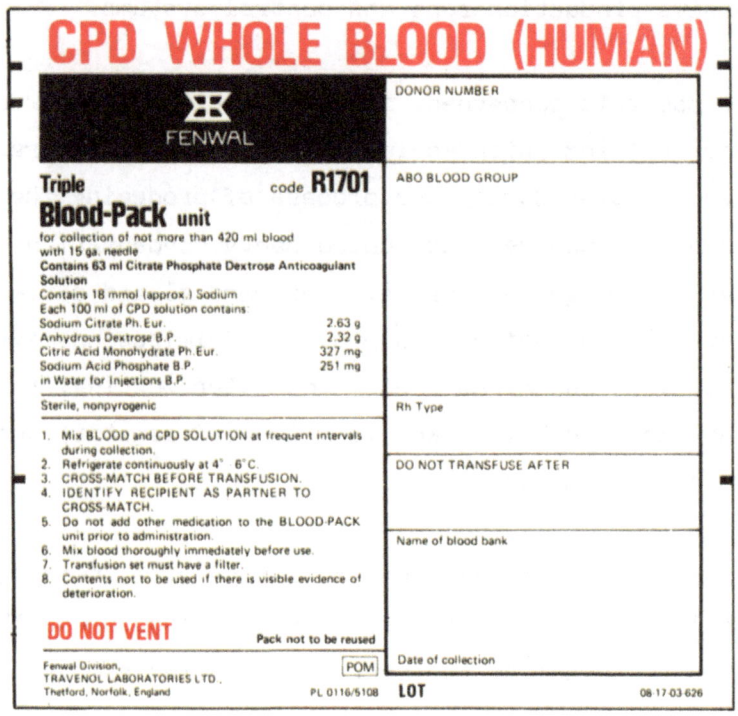

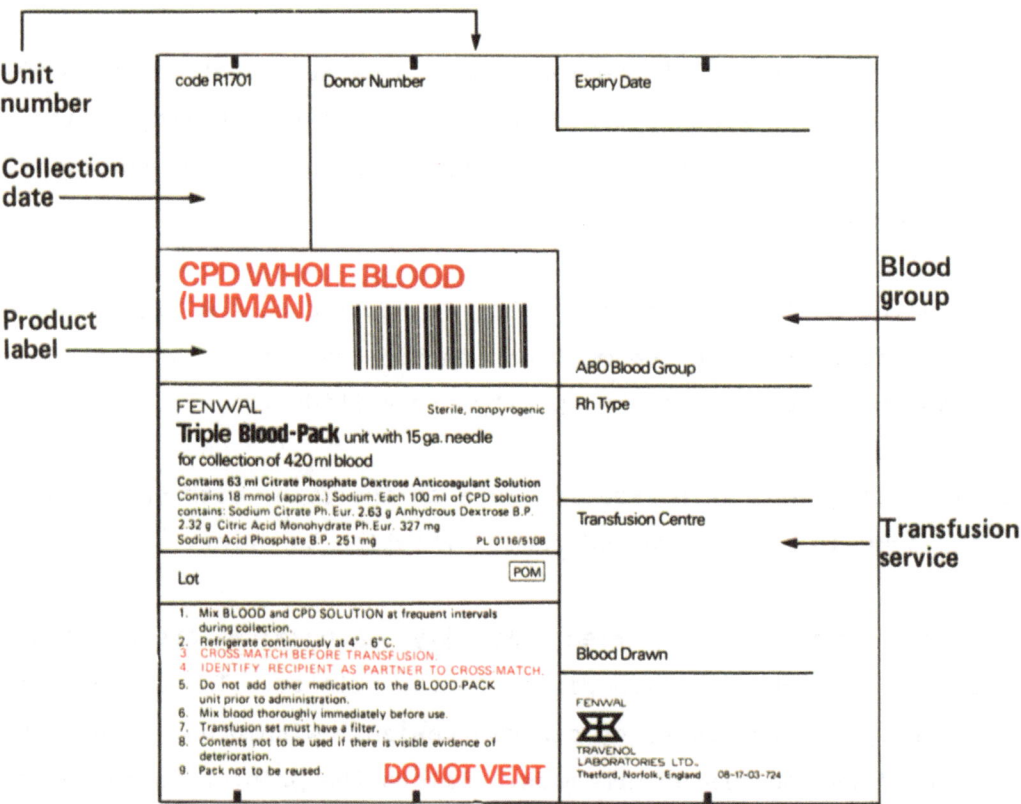

The uppermost label is the conventional, familiar label. The lower label is the label which we are now applying to our single double and triple packs.

At this stage, the same basic information is found on both labels. The product title is given fuller emphasis than initially in our older label and it is also duplicated by the Codabar symbol. This information is in red on the labels. We were advised by the Working Party that this is preferable from their point of view.

In order to make available additional area on the labels for the positioning of additive labels, the information which refers to the anti-cogaulant formulation and directions for use of the product have been condensed as far as possible.

The lot number, which used to be tucked down at the bottom of the label, has been positioned in a place where it will not be covered, or should not during normal use be covered by any overstick labels.

The solid area in the older label has obviously been precluded because if labels are affixed over a solid area the integrity of the Codabar symbol will be invalidated.

The text free areas follow the CCBBA proposals for positioning of additive labels. The collection date will be affixed below the unit number, with provision for the blood group adjacent to it. An area is provided for the addition of the transfusion centre address.

As it stands, this label has an area at the right hand bottom corner which is important to us, from the Company's point of view, because it gives our name and our address. But as far as the actual blood pack label is concerned, it can be overlabelled by centres with their own specific requirements. Ultimately we hope to achieve a label which will leave a greater area available for centres' specific information.

In co-operation with Brentwood, we have designed a range of additive overstick labels. Specifically these are the product label, additive blood product labels, and also centre specific labels depending on those centres that wish to use these labels. These are to be fully described by Mr Williams. We propose to make these labels available to those centres needing them for use with their blood packs.

The transfer pack labels have been redesigned. The layout is similar, and there should be no confusion. The only warning statement is "Do No Vent", which is in red. At the next revision of the label we shall probably also put the CPD transfer pack or the ACD transfer pack statement in red.

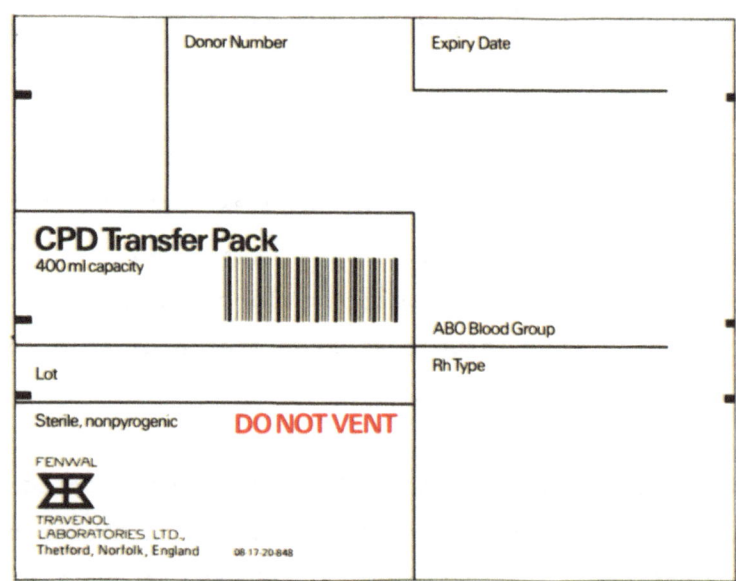

Additive labels - again labels for the transfer packs are used in the same way as the primary pack labels.

This, then, is the first stage in achieving a simplified Codabar label.

At this stage we would welcome any comments which the users may have for its improvement. It is only through use that the requirements and modifications become apparent, and it is our wish to provide the users with the label that they need rather than the label that we think they should perhaps use.

Our final goal is to achieve the ultimate simple blood pack label, which, and I quote from the CCBBA Report:

> "... contains only those items and instructions absolutely
> necessary for the proper use of the blood product. These
> items must be presented so that they are easily seen and
> clearly understood ...".

Let me now attempt to show what effect that will have on the current label. First,

> "... contains only those items and instructions absolutely
> necessary for the proper use of the blood product ..."

Are all these statements really necessary, and do they clarify or confuse?

-       "Mix blood and CPD solution at frequent intervals
        during collection."

-       "Refrigerate continuously at 4⁰ - 6⁰ Centigrade".

Two sentences in capital letters printed in red:-

        "Crossmatch before transfusion."

-       "Identify recipient as partner to crossmatch."   Then,

-       "Do not add other medication to blood pack unit
        prior to administration."

-       "Mix blood thoroughly immediately before use."

-       "Transfusion set must have a filter." What sort of filter?

- "Contents not to be used if there is visible evidence
  of deterioration."

- "Pack not to be re-used."

Obviously there will be discussion as to which of these statements are
essential. We should like to be able to present users with a label in
which all the information that is essential could be enclosed in the smallest
area possible so that the lower half of the label would be available for use by
the specific information at the centres.

The statement:
- "Fenwal triple blood pack with 15 gauge needle for
  collection of 420 ml blood,".

and the statement giving the anti-coagulant formulation; are these entirely
necessary on blood pack labels?

In order to achieve the final simplified label, we shall have to have some
guidance on what is acceptable, and not only from the users themselves. It will
involve discussions with the Department of Health, and the British Standards
Institution.

We shall be discussing these proposals ourselves with the Working Party and the
departments concerned, together with another proposal to label our anti-coagulant
solution to conform with the 1978 Addendum to the British Pharmacopoeia. This
involves the adjustment of volumes. I believe that the volumes that we are
quoting for the anti-coagulant solution have grown up historically, but we should
like some guidance on users' feelings about this.

If and when agreement is reached on the further simplified label, we would
undertake at Travenol to supply blood packs so labelled as and when the Regional
Transfusion Centres are ready to accept them.

We have prepared a manual which aims to explain and illustrate the labelling
changes which have been described. This manual includes a final artist's
impression of the simplified label on which we would like to form our initial
proposals. Copies of the manual are available to all at this meeting. It

includes a presentation of the labelled blood bag and comparisons of the existing labelling for the codes which are now labelled with the Codabar labels, as well as a rather cunning little presentation of a label which has been overlabelled with additive labels and our artist's impressions of the final Codabar simplified label.

We shall be sending out additional pages to add to this manual illustrating fully the overstick labels which we hope to supply with the blood bags.

As any changes or additions to our labels are made, we shall also send our further sheets to be included in the file so that information can be kept up to date.

EXPERIENCE WITH MACHINE READABLE LABELS
AT THE NEW YORK BLOOD CENTER
Dr E Brodeim

It is a pleasure for me to be here participating in this Meeting. I shall say
something about the characteristic of Codabar and describe how we are using it
at The New York Blood Center.

We have now worked with Codabar for several years. During this time we have made
progress, primarily on the basis of trial and error, with certain concepts for
using computers in conjunction with bar codes.

Properties of Bar Codes

The use of bar code provides a system that is not susceptible to clerical errors
that can result in the transfusion of wrong blood units. The particular bar
code, Codabar, was selected for a number of reasons. In Codabar the possibility
of one character being read as another is extremely small. Although we can use
the 7 binary digits of the Codabar code to represent 128 different characters,
it has been restricted to only 20 characters.

These 20 characters have been selected very carefully so that no single
replacement of a wide bar by a narrow bar or a wide space by a narrow space (or
vice versa) can result in the wrong character being represented. In most
cases, even two bits being transposed through this type of error will not result
in another character being represented. The number of one character substitution
per 1 million reads was an upper limit in our design. We have read over 1 million
unit number labels on blood units on our GROUPAMATICS and have yet to find a
transposition error. So we can safely say that the substitution rate is an
extremely small number.

Another important characteristic of this symbol is that because of this high
redundancy all of the checking is done on a character-by-character basis. We do
not depend on word parity in the machine-readable form. This is important because
in the progressive labelling of a blood product, we have to keep appending
information, so the size of the message will merely start with a unit number.
Added to this is the collection date identification. Subsequently a blood type
identification label is added so the size of the word keeps changing. Any symbol
that depends on the security of having a word parity would not work in this
environment because the length of the word keeps changing. A symbol that has
parity controlled on a character-by-character basis provides that kind of
flexibility.

When the Committee for Commonality in Blood Banking Automation was formed in the US, one of the primary motivating factors was that there was a great deal of interest in automation, and many very inventive researchers were inventing very many symbols, all of which had some desirable characteristics. We were very rapidly getting to the point when, in the foreseeable future, we would have as many different symbols used in blood banking as we have inventive researchers - of whom we were graced by quite a large number. Fortunately, we managed to persuade all of these people to pool their talents on what became the Committee for Commonality in Blood Banking Automation. Perhaps the largest measure of the success of this group is that to the very best of our knowledge, all of the automation efforts at this time in the US are based on the use of this symbol. This involved many researchers backtracking on their own cherished inventions of many years, not forgetting one of my own colleagues, Hal Allan, as well as Bob Chambers then of Georgetown University, and many others, all of whom had spent quite a deal of time in developing different symbol approaches. It is greatly to their credit that they were able to subvert their personal interests to the common interest in blood banking.

The symbol is merely a tool for representing information. It does not in any way impinge upon the ingenuity with which it is applied. We now have the added gratification of seeing many other transfusion services, including that of the United Kingdom, consider this symbol. It is an extremely nice outcome.

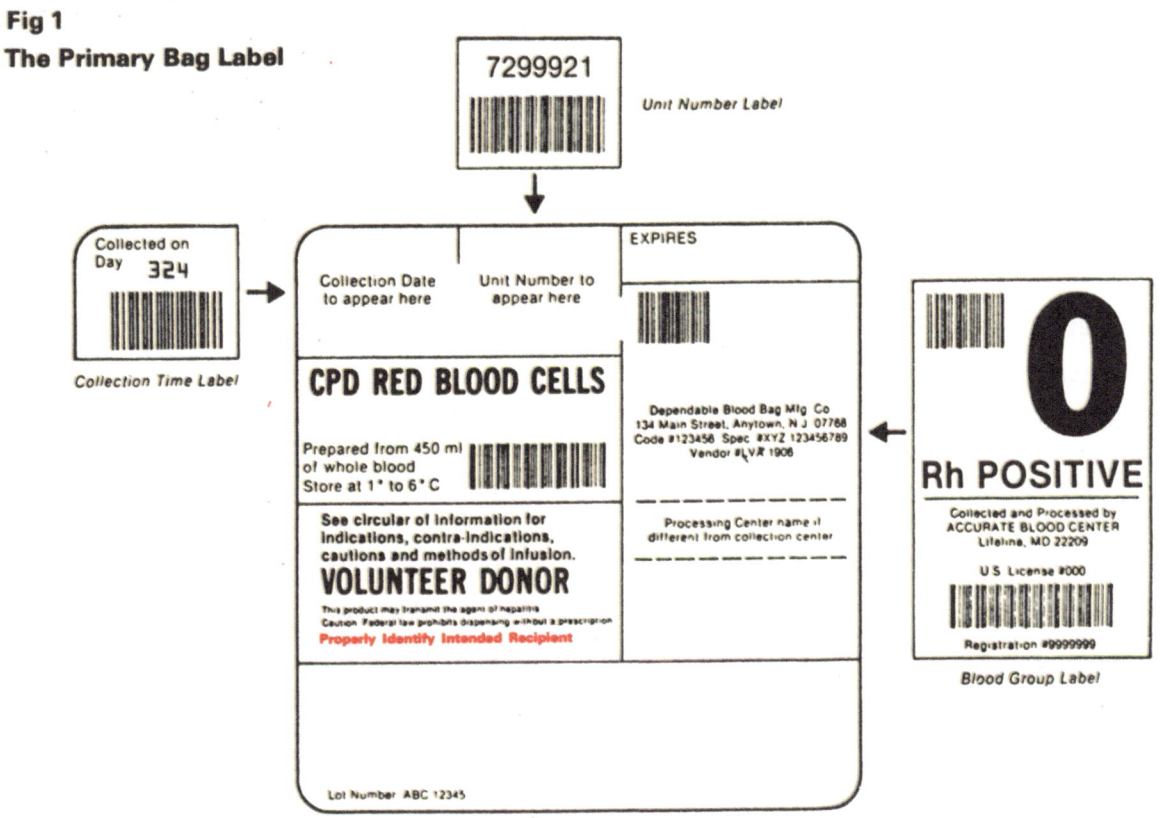

Fig 1
The Primary Bag Label

21

Let me outline some of the applications of the symbol and how we are proposing to use it.

The proposed US primary bag label, which is to be published in the Federal Register in the US, is very similar to the label which was published in the Final Report of the Commonality Committee. A few minor changes have been made to its wording, but not to the representation of the machine-readable code. The bag label has been divided into clearly defined areas for the unit number, for the collection date, for information concerning who processed it and who collected it, and even provision for both pieces of information to be shown when one centre collects and another centre processes. An area has been reserved for whatever general instructions need to be conveyed, the primary part being a message to see a circular of information for indications, contra-indications, cautions and methods of infusion. One interesting by-product is that for the first time in the United States we have a common circle of information on which the three blood-banking organisations have worked together. A US peculiarity is that our law requires each unit to be labelled whether it comes from a volunteer donor or from a paid donor. We also require a warning that the product may transmit agents of hepatitis and that Federal Law prohibits dispensing without a prescription. These are required by law. Almost everyone agrees that they should not be there, so we have put them in print that is rather hard to see. On the other hand, the caution to properly identify the intended recipient was felt to be important and consequently is prominently displayed in red.

The placement of machine readable information, of the collection date, the unit number and the blood type area was selected for a number of reasons. As Mrs Jackson pointed out, we want to force people to read the unit number and the blood type as a single message. This is perhaps the most important association - that this unit is that blood type. The protocol can require that these messages must be read as one. However, only if these labels are next to each other on the same label is it possible to make that read. We feel that is a very important safety feature.

Let me point out one particular bar code. The bar code to the right of the unit number area says that this would be a CPD bag with, say, two satellite packs to it. The reason for that is worth considering. Only the unit number label and that code will appear on it when the unit is brought back to the blood centre. A log-in process will read that unit number and the type of bag to which that unit number corresponds. The example shown opposite means that unit 7299921 is a CPD triple pack. Having this information read into the computer as soon as the unit is brought in is really the start of the laboratory's production control, because this shows how many singles, how many doubles and how many triples are in processing. It is the starting point of being able to decide whether there are enough platelets to be made, etc. It is an important code to put on. In adapting this label to different countries, the language of the eye-readable information will change. The proposed Travenol pack which was shown earlier is a very nice example of adapting it to a particular situation - as in the United Kingdom - while maintaining the integrity of the machine readable information. But, one thing I should like to suggest for Travenol's consideration is the inclusion of the bag bar code which I just discussed which will come in useful further on.

I should also like to point out that the area at the bottom of the label that has been left blank has been left blank for a reason. Eventually it is intended to provide room for associating the unit number with the identification of the intended recipient.

In making the design we have tried to think all the time of having bedside verification as the ultimate step to ensure that the proper product is transfused to the proper recipient. This area has been reserved for machine-readable labels that will facilitate that.

Fig 2 The Satellite Bag Label

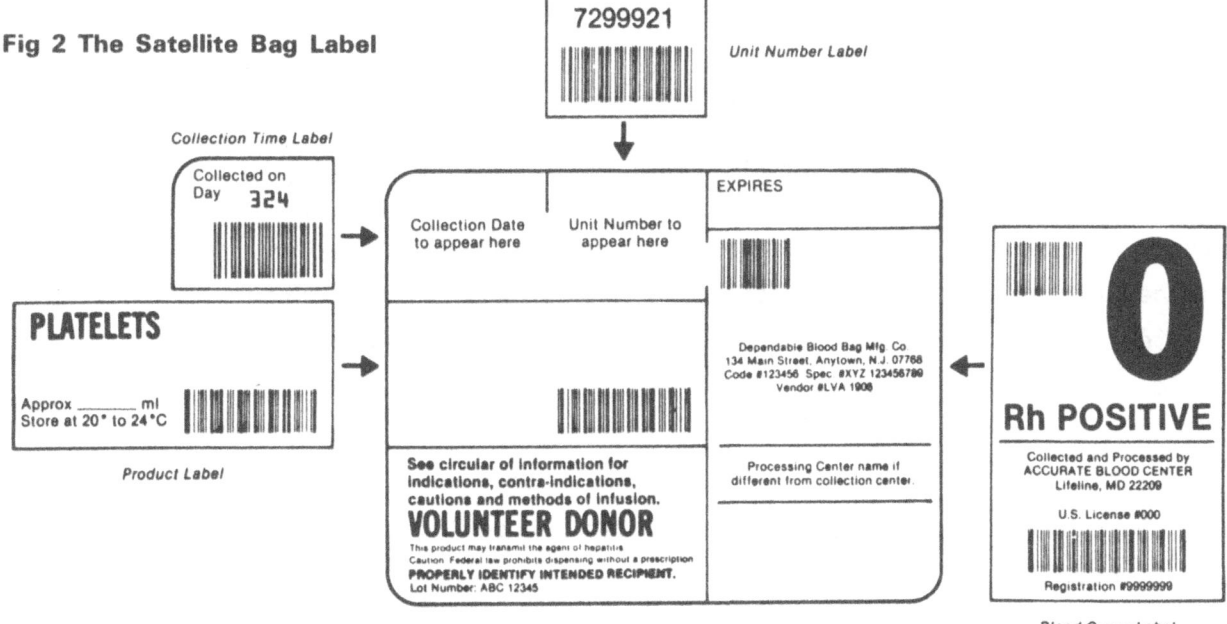

The satellite pack labels are very similar in design. The space at the bottom for the recipient linkage is omitted only because there is no room for it and there is probably less need for it on a satellite pack. Since we do not know what the product is, the product area is left to be labelled by whatever component is made, in this case platelets. We should note that an empty pack is also given a product code, since in the production control systems, such as the one we are implementing in New York, if a triple pack is received, each part of the triple pack must be accounted for. If one winds up sending an empty satellite along with the primary pack, for example for pediatric use, that is fine, but the empty pack must be scanned out when it is shipped so that there is accountability for each part of every blood bag. Other than that, the label is very much the same as on the primary bag.

Range of Applications

Let us now take a look at some of the applications of bar codes.

Fig 3   Bar Code Use In Blood Donor-Recipient Linkage System

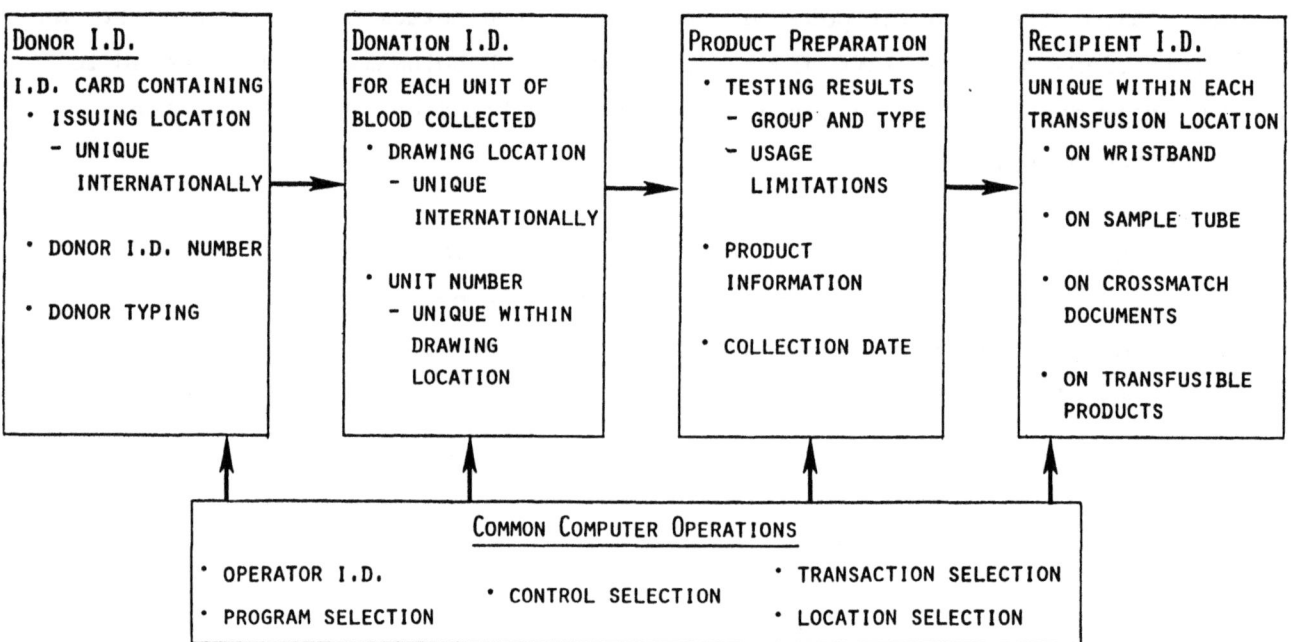

The range of applications that we had in mind when machine readable codes were introduced had as the first step the identification of a blood donor. It was postulated that blood donor identification cards could contain, in machine-readable form:-

-   the issuing location; which of the centres in, for example, the United Kingdom or the United States issued it. This would be a number that is internationally unique.

-   a donor identification number assigned by the centre so that the combination of this number with the above would also be internationally unique.

-   possibly some information about the donor's previous typing.

24

For each blood donation there is provision on the pack label to show the drawing location, which is - as was pointed out - internationally unique. All drawing locations in the United States start with a digit '5'. Those in the United Kingdom would start with a digit '7', and so on. In addition, a unique number is assigned to each donation by each blood centre. In the United States that number is required to be unique for a period of five years. In the preparation of the product we provide for the addition of the group and type, or a usage limitation. For example, a unit may not be suitable for transfusion and would have to be so labelled.

The label will also show the particular product that is in the bag and the collection date. The combination of a product code and collection date is equivalent to and is translated by the computer into an expiration date. The reason why we use collection dates and not expiration dates is that at the time the unit is collected we did not know what might go into each of the satellite packs.

For the recipient we have postulated the use of a machine-readable identification on each recipient's wristband, which could also be in machine-readable form. That same number will be transferred to the patient's sample tube on transfusion request or cross-match documents that are maintained by the blood bank. That number will eventually be transferred to the blank area at the bottom of the blood pack so that final verification can take place at the patient's bedside that the product that is about to be transfused is properly suited to that patient.

Bar codes are also extensively used in the control of the computer operations at the blood centre, and they can also be used within the hospital blood bank. They are used for the identification of the person who is responsible for an operation, who is usually the person who is entering the information into the computer; for the selection of the particular operation that is being done, the labelling of blood or what have you; for identification of where it is to be shipped to, and so on. The intent of all of this is to make the automation of data entry a totally bar code driven operation. In other words, the objective is to do away with the traditional keyboard as the means for entering or capturing information, and to make all information capture operations strictly a bar code reading operation.

Status of Implementation
Before looking at the mechanics of this, let me briefly identify how far along we are in each of the operations.

Fig 4

<u>STATUS OF BAR CODE APPLICATION</u>

<u>IN</u>

<u>BLOOD BANKING AUTOMATION</u>

. DONOR IDENTIFICATION
   - CONCEPTUAL DESIGN

. DONATION IDENTIFICATION
   - FULLY DEVELOPED BY CCBBA

. PRODUCT PREPARATION
   - FULLY DEVELOPED BY CCBBA

. RECIPIENT IDENTIFICATION
   - RESEARCH PROPOSAL

. COMMON COMPUTER OPERATIONS
   - EXPERIMENTAL DEVELOPMENT
     AT THE NEW YORK BLOOD
     CENTER

On donor identification, we got as far as the conceptual design. We had a
funding cut for the Commonality Committee and we had to disband the task force
before a final recommendation was made. The donation identification and the
product preparation recommendations were finished by the Commonality Committee,
and are contained in the final report - as Mrs Jackson pointed out. A recipient
identification system was taken through the conceptual phase by the Commonality
Committee. We have a research proposal in from the New York Blood Center, in
which I am participating with some other colleagues, for making a prototype of a
recipient linkage that will be compatible with the work already done.

The computer operations are being driven at the New York Blood Center strictly by
bar code. Mrs Jackson has already mentioned much of this.

Any bar code such as the product code for platelets for example, are made up in three parts.

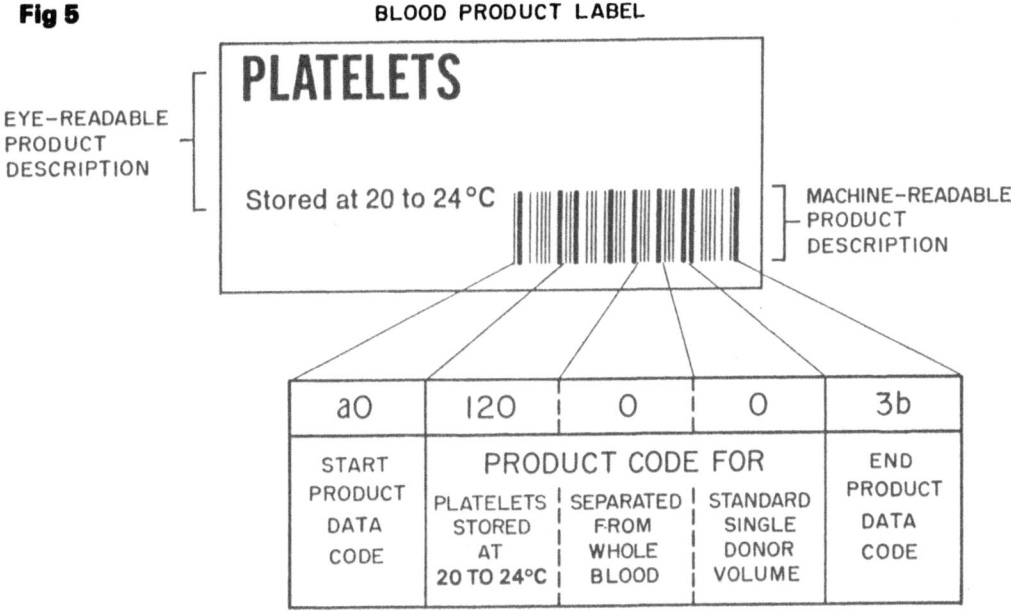

Fig 5

BLOOD PRODUCT LABEL

EYE-READABLE PRODUCT DESCRIPTION

PLATELETS

Stored at 20 to 24°C

MACHINE-READABLE PRODUCT DESCRIPTION

a0	120	0	0	3b
START PRODUCT DATA CODE	PRODUCT CODE FOR			END PRODUCT DATA CODE
	PLATELETS STORED AT 20 TO 24°C	SEPARATED FROM WHOLE BLOOD	STANDARD SINGLE DONOR VOLUME	

The product information, or whatever the information is, is embedded between two sets of control codes. The first three digits of the product code explain what the product is; in this case platelets stored at 20° - 24°C. The next digit identifies it as being obtained from whole blood as opposed to pheresis. The last digit identifies it as standard single donor volume.

These control codes do two things. First, they are necessary for the light pen to read something. The light pen logic requires a start/stop character at each end of the bar codes that tells it which way it is reading the code. We went from the traditional single character start/stop code to two character control code right at the beginning, for a very important reason. We wanted each of the combinations of control codes to be unique within the entire range of blood banking applications. Unique codes have been reserved all the way through recipient identification. There is an important reason for this. Much of the problem with the use of computers lies in the old saying "garbage in, garbage out". Whenever information is keyed into a computer, the problem lies in being able to control that what is entered is accurate. Once inaccurate data is entered into the computer, it can sometimes be such a pain in the neck to track it down and purge it from the system that whatever advantages may have been gained by automation are lost, and with interest, in trying to clean out the garbage. A chief advantage of bar codes is really that if the data is entered then it is entered accurately; otherwise it is not entered at all. It is virtually impossible, if a proper protocol is used, to get wrong data in. That is in part because of the security that these control codes provide. If this is

programmed properly, then when the computer expects a product code it must start
and end with the proper control codes. Further, it must have precisely five
characters in between the control codes which must match up the list of
possibilities.

To cut a long story short. When something is entered with a light pen, if the
bar codes are readable at all it must enter the correct information. One
cannot, for example, accidentally enter an identification number instead of a
product code even if the data part of it is the same, because the control codes
will catch it. Two characters cannot be transposed. In fact, no wrong information
can be entered at all. If some thought is given to the cost of writing computer
programs, most of the cost and the difficulty, and the potential user
dissatisfaction is related to the fact that it is possible to get wrong data in.
The key is to set up the system not to permit the wrong data to get in in the
first place, rather than to clean it out when it does. This is really the main
advantage of using machine-readable codes as opposed to the conventional methods
of getting data into computers and it is why we have gone to very considerable
lengths to use light-pen data entry as the method of entry, not only for the
identification of things dealing with blood samples, but for all computer
operations.

Flexibility of Bar Code System

Another item that I want to touch on briefly concerns the flexibility that this
particular bar code system provides. Mrs Jackson has pointed out that the code
'd' is a special code. It can either be used to indicate the start of a
message or the break between two messages that are to be considered as one.

Fig 6   **BLOOD UNIT LABEL**

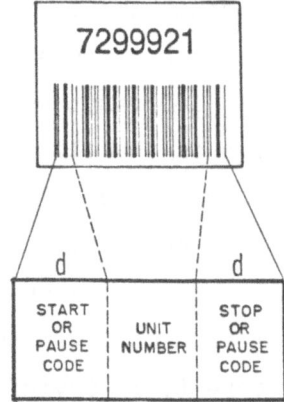

The unit number has a 'd' at the start and at the end because this bar code could
be embedded between codes on both sides of it. Another very pragmatic reason why
we had to use only a single control code around the unit number is not quite as
profound. On the GROUPAMATIC, the way the device is constructed there is only

28

room for nine characters, otherwise the holder obscures some of the characters. Initially this meant that it had to be kept down to nine, and since it had to be kept down to nine this was the one piece of information we chose to put in the middle of the other pieces.

Fig 7

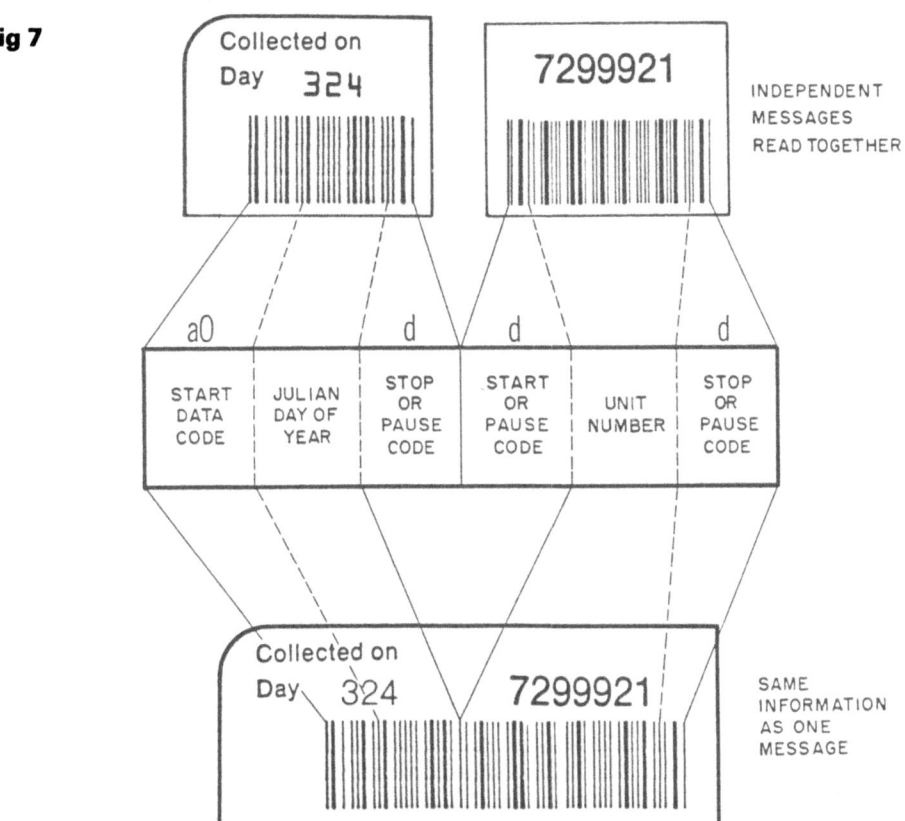

This diagram shows how it works. On the blood bag, for example, the collection date bar code can be put in the top left hand corner. The unit number bar code is then placed next to it and the blood type bar code will be right next to it on the other side. The collection date bar code starts with the control code 'AO'. It has the Julian day of the year which is just a count from 1 to 365, followed by a pause code. The unit number label starts with a pause code, is followed by the unit number and ends with another pause code. When a light pen is run across both labels then the two adjacent pause codes cancel each other out and we are left with the start code, the Julian day, the unit number and the 'd' stop code. If a transfusion centre is set up so that blood can be collected at fixed sites, then it is possible to combine the collection date label and the unit number label into a single label that provides both the collection date and the unit number. It can be printed as a single label instead of the two stick-on labels to be put on at different times.

The system gives the flexibility of combining messages. Thus there is flexibility in how the information goes on the bag. We ourselves were very concerned with not having the tail wag the dog, so to speak, having the peculiarities of the

bar code restrict how a particular blood centre could operate, and with providing
the flexibility to let each blood centre operate as it wished; but provided that
all fully labeled bags should look identical to a bar code reader.

Application to Computer Operations

Bar codes are used to identify persons, programs and hospitals to which a centre
might ship blood. The Hospital Selection Sheet gives the names and the addresses
of all of the hospitals to which the Long Island Blood Centre ships blood with
the bar code next to each of them.

Fig 8

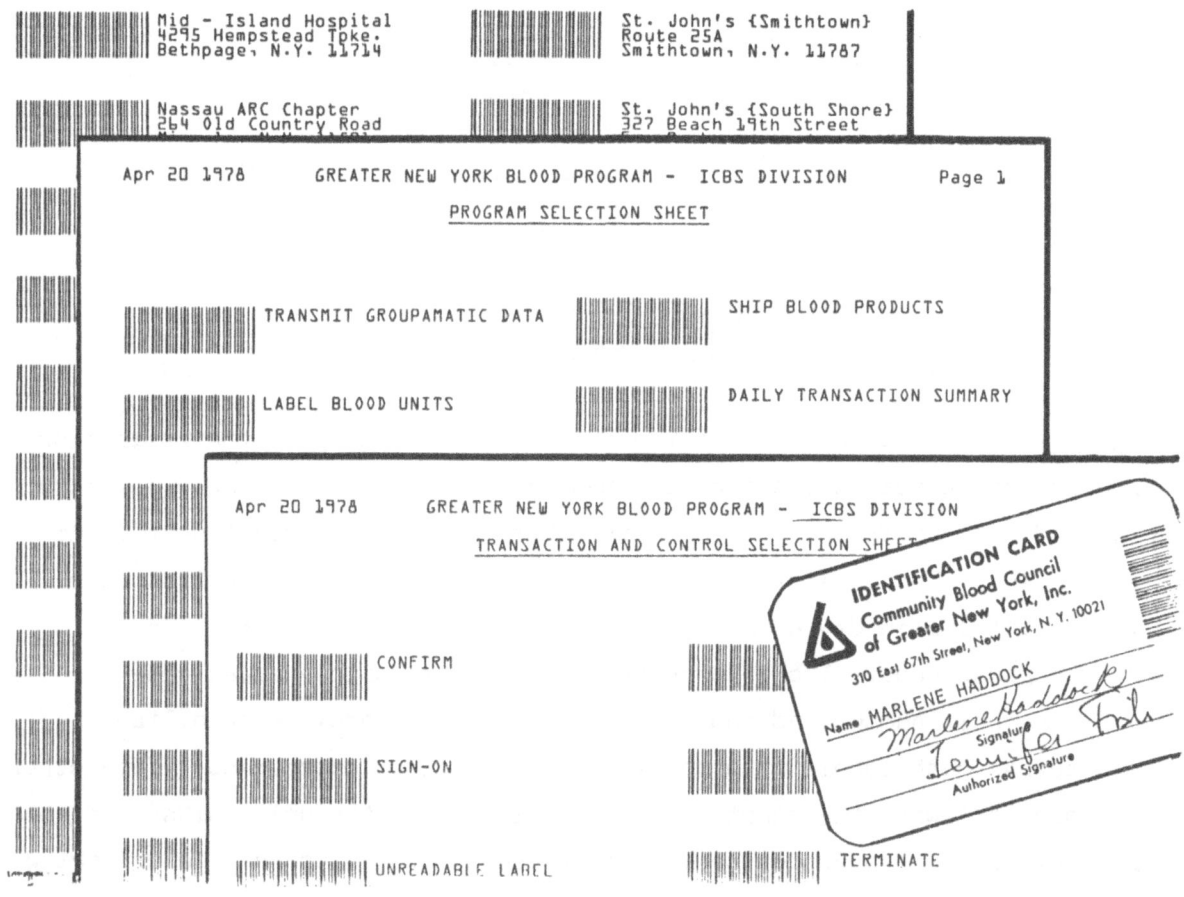

To designate, say, the St John's South Shore Hospital one would merely scan the
correct bar code. The computer could recognise from the control code that this
is a hospital, and out from the data part of it which particular hospital it is.

To select a particular program to be run, eg to transmit GROUPAMATIC data from one site to another or to label blood products, you scan the appropriate bar code on the Program Selection Sheet. In order to get on to the computer in the first place one would have to identify oneself, which is done by scanning a bar code on the identification cards that are issued to all employees. The computer will look up who it is and then see if that person has any business running the program they are trying to run. Assuming that that is the case, it will put the name on the screen, let that program be run and hold the person running it responsible for whatever is done.

That means that it is possible to track every unit of blood back, find out who was responsible for logging it into the blood centre, who separated it into components, who was responsible for each test that was performed, who labelled it, who shipped it, and when. In short we set up a complete audit trail.

There are further bar code functions provided for. If a label is unreadable the non-readable bar code label can be scanned, and one is allowed to key in the number on an exception principle and so on. In effect, every operation is initiated by the scanning of a bar and in no case is a keying in of any information required on a routine basis.

If the program that has been selected by scanning from the program select sheet is to ship blood, then the destination to which the blood is to be shipped is specified by scanning from the hospital selection sheet. The bar codes on the units to be shipped are then scanned. The transaction is terminated by scanning a terminate code on the control sheet. There is a complete sequence of bar code scans that controls the entire operation from beginning to end. I shall not go through all the logical paths but they are fairly self-evident.

Logical Automation Flow

A very simplified representation of how we should have gone about automation is shown here. We actually started by automating the blood processing, and we did this for historical reasons. Dr Jenkins pointed out that the punched card sample identification system on the GROUPAMATIC is totally unsatisfactory.

Fig 9

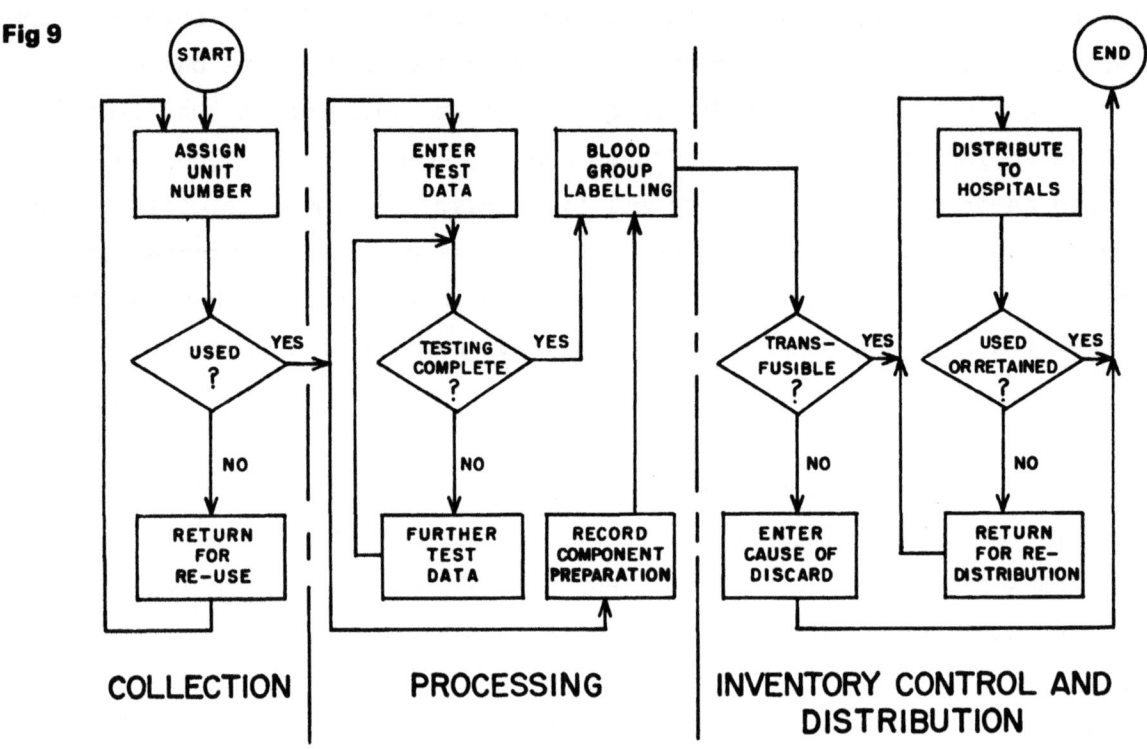

We developed the laser system as a substitute for it and it was subsequently used by KONTRON on all of such units. We had pressing reasons for starting with the blood processing, and it is a pressing set of reasons that I have regretted ever since the day we did it.

Unfortunately, blood processing is right in the middle of the logical flow. That logical flow really starts when blood unit identification numbers are assigned to a collection site. They are either used, or they are returned, in which case they can be logged back in. Once the units are used, then some test data has to be entered from them. A check is set up to determine if all testing is complete. If it is not then further test data will have to be enetered until it is. Concurrently the blood units will be broken into components and the components being produced must be recorded. Each of the components must then be labelled to agree with the testing that was done. If these units are transfusable they can be sent out. If not, one will have to say why one is getting rid of them so as to account for them. If they are sent out, they may not be used by the hospital. In that case they may be returned for redistribution and will go back into the loop. It is a very logical flow from beginning to end.

If one does not start from the beginning of this flow - as we did not - then one really has a problem. We, for example, picked up units as they were tested on the GROUPAMATIC. We had absolutely no idea, and we still have no prior idea of what units will come through on the GROUPAMATIC.

We have a difficult time accounting for units that somehow get lost between being assigned and coming back on the GROUPAMATIC, and we are forever merging together information and all kinds of havoc result as a consequence.

What I am really getting at is this: there is a logical starting place. Certainly if I had to do it over again I would not dream of starting anywhere but at the logical beginning.

If one does start at the beginning, then it really becomes a very straightforward situation. There will be unit numbers issued to collection sites. One finds out a steadily increasing amount of information about the unit numbers as one goes on. As one gets test results they are associated with unit numbers; as components are labelled and as they are distributed, etc further data is added. It becomes a matter of updating more and more information about known quantities. If one fails to do this, one will keep getting surprises. Units will pop out of nowhere. We all know how units are supposed to be processed. The problem is that it does not work that way. A couple of them, for some reason, will get taken out of the rack and will not appear with the rest of their colleagues but will appear a day later, and so on. Such things may sound trivial but they can cause quite a bit of havoc.

Summary

By way of summary, the bar code and the methods for its reading have held up very well. The bar code does all of the things that it was supposed to do. It is highly readable. It is highly flexible. The equipment for reading is reliable. The original lasers on the GROUPAMATIC are still functioning after two years. We have read upwards of a million and a half samples with them. We read better than 99 per cent of all the labels. We have not had a single substitution error.

The light pen used for driving automation has also held up very well. It is very easy to learn how to use light pens. Clerical level people can learn how to use them very quickly. They can use them very accurately. In fact, they use them a lot better than researchers were ever able to do. I cannot achieve the same flexibility or the same speed as the people in the shipping department have achieved. We now use it for all laboratory functions and all distribution functions, and we hope we shall soon be moving back to fill up that hole in the collection area.

One of the technological problems has been that the development of the equipment for printing bar codes has not moved as fast as we had hoped that it would. There are now very important breakthroughs coming, not so much because we have triggered them in blood banking, but because the use of bar codes in the supermarkets is finally taking off in the United States. Because of that, the manufacturers are really pushing printing devices.

One of the things that we have to recognise is that in blood banking we can take advantage of technological trends, but we really cannot set them. We are not an important enough market segment for manufacturers to undertake the rather extensive development cost to make the new technology available. One of the reasons we went for the bar code was the mistaken belief, two years ago, that they were about to take off in large quantitites in the supermarkets. There were some system problems that were peculiar to the supermarkets that delayed it, but I think that these have finally been solved. We hope to be getting a prototype of a bar code printer to be used in the blood centre in the very near future, and we shall start to make our own bar code labels. We need to perfect labels that are not vulnerable to smearing or to any of the other problems that arise in the rather hostile environment (to the labels) of blood banking.

The control of the print quality, to which Travenol has alluded, is also a real problem. Sensible devices that really check the print quality are only now coming on to the market: rapid speed lasers that will rapidly read a large number of times and give a quantitative measure of how well a particular bar code reads.

Lasers have come in a long way. The difficulty has been that the lasers that we used on the GROUPAMATIC were really the first inexpensive laser devices made. We paid for the lack of expense by sacrificing a great deal in depth of field - which we did not need on the GROUPAMATIC. But these devices are not suitable for such applications as shipping. We are now able to have lasers which have a much broader field of view and which are much more compact. We hope to have an experimental unit working in the shipping department - probably within the next thirty days - when it should no longer be necessary to teach people how to wave a light pen. It will only be necessary to bring a blood bag into the quite wide field of view of the laser to enter data in. So there are some continued technological developments.

Another major area is a recognition of how the programming for automation should proceed. There are two schools of thought about programming. One, adopted by our colleagues at KONTRON says "tell us the problems, we shall understand them and we shall provide you with the programs that do the things you want to do". There is an advantage to this in the sense that the manufacturer, at least, takes full responsibility. But to my mind there is a major disadvantage. Any change, no matter how trivial, has to go back to the software people, and in my opinion that is not an acceptable situation. Blood banking is far too fluid a field for that approach to work.

The approach that we have taken is to let the programmers devise a very flexible framework in which the blood bankers will do the final programming. Let me give an example of what I mean by this. The labelling of blood products can be viewed as a two-step process. We do a number of tests which between them establish the ABO, and we do further tests which establish the Rh. We may have one or more tests designed to determine if untoward antibodies are present, and so on. We look at it as a process whereby there are a number of basic tests from which intermediate results such as ABO and Rh are formed. How the blood product is labelled is a function of what combinations of intermediate results are required to label a product in a certain way. For example, for a unit to be labelled A-positive it must be Group A, it must be Rh positive, it must be negative for antibody, it must be negative for hepatitis, and so on. Then it can be labelled Group A positive. The framework is the two matrices one of which translates the basic test to the intermediate results, and another which translates combinations of intermediate results to a labelling state.

A laboratory director can be trained to enter the logic for the matrix, and to modify it if a new test is to be incorporated or for whatever reason the logic of labelling is to be changed. This is the key in my opinion, but it is hindsight, and not the way the original programs were developed. It is the way we are developing them now. It is important, in my opinion, not to give the total responsibility to computer people. The final logic has to be designed so that the people who understand blood banking can understand it and can do it. This requires a fair amount of understanding, but it can be done, and I believe very firmly that it is the way that it should be done.

Let me say again that I appreciate the opportunity to be here and to share our experiences in this application.

Questions to Dr BRODHEIM
========================

Prof STRATTON (Manchester): It seems to me from what has been said here that
the object of the identification number is to get the fewest number of digits
with the maximum variation so that people can understand it easily when it is
written out. Car registration plates, bank notes, airline tickets, or anything
one can think of have a combination of numerals and letters. Why has a
combination of numerals and letters not been used for bar codes? This would
give greater variation with fewer digits than numerals alone.

Dr BRODHEIM: It is a good question and there are two reason for it. By going
to an all-numeric system and only providing a limited number of special
characters we are able to embed a very high degree of redundancy in the code.
We have a basic problem. The size of a blood bag is relatively small for the
amount of information that has to be placed on it. What basically limits the
size of the printing of any machine-readable code is the resolution that is
required to get the smallest bar. If, then, the attitude is one of wanting a
code with a very high degree of redundancy, this limits the number of
characters that are available if those characters are to be printed in a finite
amount of space.

It was really a trade-off characteristic between providing the amount of
information in the space that is available and providing the highest degree
of security. It is true that if we went to an alphabetic character set, or
an alpha-numeric character set, we would need fewer characters to convey the
same information, but in order to provide the same security into this much
larger character set, we would have to make each character wider, and the
trade-off in the opinion of our symbol selection task force was to go to an all-
numberic number set.

I should make one addendum to this. Since many blood banks, at least in the
United States, have a long standing tradition of using alphabetical characters
to distinguish between mobile collection units, there is a provision for
translating what is really a strictly numerical character set into an eye-readable
alphanumerical character set. The Commonality Committee Report has a proposed
translation table for three numberic characters to be represented by two
alphabetical characaters in the eye-readable form. So this means blood centres
can continue their longstanding practices of using alphanumerical character sets.

The specific answer to the question is that viewing the need for redundancy and security, it was the feeling of the symbol selection task force that it was better achieved by a more limited character set rather than going to the wider character set. Looking at single-digit transpositions and what they could transpose into, the larger the character set, the more the probability goes up, and it does not go up in a linear manner but almost on the square of the number of characters. Keeping the number of characters to the smallest number possible will also provide the highest level of security.

Prof STRATTON: Is Dr Brodheim saying that the number of bars needed to represent a letter is greater than the number of bars needed to represent a numeral?

Dr BRODHEIM: Absolutely.

There is a variant of Codabar, Code 39, which is a full alphanumeric character set, and it was considered. What it has is a fifth bar. The fifth bar will extend Codabar to a full alphanumeric character set.

Prof STRATTON: But with the numbers the blood centres are likely to use, which I take to be about ten million, any number may reproduce within a year.

Dr BRODHEIM: The unit number itself does not have to be unique. The combination of the unit number and the centre number have to be unique.

That is how we get around the problem. In other words, the 7-digit number must not repeat at one collection centre. However, the same unit number can be used at different collection centres because they are distinguished by the centre identification number.

Dr JENKINS: In fact some members of our Working Party would like to reduce the eye-readable number to six digits for hospital use. By using the centre identification code, we can run for eight years without repeats, even on the six-digit, for the average centre in the UK.

Dr BRODHEIM: I am glad that Dr Jenkins brought that point up. The protocol also says that leading Zeros in bar codes are not printed in eye-readable form. For the smaller collection centre the number can be reduced to six digits, to five digits or even to four digits in eye-readable form, because the leading Zeros do not print.

Dr NAPIER (Cardiff): As blood banks start to exploit the possibilities for computerisation of inventory control and blood product issues, bar codes will be needed for extra jobs, and the control or start-stop codes will have to be selected for this. Is it desirable to achieve uniformity in the use of control codes, or are the individual centres to be free to select their own control codes?

Dr BRODHEIM: It all depends on the specific application. One set of control codes had been reserved for what we call local use. In other words, every centre can use these for whatever purposes it sees fit. However, for anything that has broad application, we have set up through the ISBT Working Party on Automation a mechanism where the Secretary of ISBT, the Chairman of the Council of Europe Expert Group, and the Chairman of the Technical Advisory Panel of the American Blood Commission will co-ordinate the assignment of new control codes as required. It is necessary to distinguish whether the application is peculiar to the centre, in which it is suggested that the control codes that have been set aside for that purpose should be used, or whether this is something that would be usable by other centres, in which case I would strongly urge that the ISBT mechanism for having these assigned be used.

Dr JENKINS: In the UK we want to encourage people to use the existing Working Party because there is a link between the Working Party and the ISBT. We have two members who are also members of ISBT, and the Secretary can communicate directly with the Chairman of the appropriate committee of ISBT. If ISBT is not interested, and if it is a local problem, then I would like to think that the National Working Party can award the codes and know what anybody is using at any time.

Dr CASH (Scotland): Dr Brodheim talked about digit numbers and said that it was possible to get down to five, or maybe four, depending on collection size. May I

ask Dr Brodheim what a 4 digit versus a 7 digit difference means in relation
to collection size?

Dr BRODHEIM: I do not know what the requirements in the UK are. In the US the
requirement is that the numbers do not reappear within a five-year period, and
it is just a matter of estimating the anticipated collections over five years and
providing enough leeway for it not to repeat. The United States still has a
large number of hospitals that run their own collection programme, or very
small blood centres - those that collect fewer than 10,000 units/year, and they
use 4-digit numbers. Most of the other centres, to the best of my knowledge,
use 7-digit numbers, although I believe that a few do use 6-digit numbers.

Dr IBBOTSON (Birmingham): We have decided to put a check digit on the end of
our 7-digit identification. We do it because we feel we may be having to key in
certain amounts of information. From what Dr Brodheim has said, it seems
desirable to go away from this.

Dr BRODHEIM: I was talking strictly about machine-readable information. It was
recommended that where a substantial amount of keying is to be done, then a check
digit should be used, but only on the eye-readable portion and placed at the end
of the number as has been suggested. In keying, a very frequent source of error
is the transposition of digits, which the software will not always catch. The
use of a modular-11 check digit, which is suggested in the Commonality
Committee Report, is a very efficient way of catching such transposition and
other common types of keying errors.

The reason why we do not use a check digit is that we have gone away completely
from the keying of these numbers. If the numbers are not keyed in, then we
believe quite strongly, on the basis of our experience, that a check digit is not
necessary. When numbers are keyed in, then I would urge that a check digit
be used.

Dr JENKINS: Are Volumes 2 and 3 readily available? Those who are actively
involved will already have copies, but other centres coming in on the scheme
should really have the Executive Volume and Volumes 2 and 3. Are they available?

Dr BRODHEIM: The American Blood Commission supposedly has copies available.
The NIH was supposed to reprint them. The first printing sold out. They are
supposed to be reprinted. In fact, all seven volumes are supposed to be
reprinted. I do not know if they are currently available. I do have a small
number of copies in reserve and I would be able to furnish a small number of copies.

REGIONAL TRANSFUSION DIRECTORS' COMMITTEE
Working Party for the Introduction of Machine-Readable Labels
INTERIM REPORT
Dr H H Gunson (Oxford Regional Transfusion Centre)

The Working Party was formed in October 1978 following an informal meeting of representatives from six Regions who had informally discussed the introduction of machine-readable labels because they had acquired automated blood grouping equipment which required the interpretation of bar-coded labels.

The terms of reference of the Working Party were:

> "To advise the Regional Transfusion Directors (RTD)
> on a satisfactory way to introduce machine-readable
> labels into the Blood Transfusion Service"

The membership of the Working Party comprised representatives from the Regional Transfusion Centres at Birmingham, Brentwood, Bristol, Edgware, Oxford and Sheffield.

It should be made clear that the Working Party has not considered computer facilities in Regional Transfusion Centres although recommendations made on the design of labels inevitably will have implications for computerisation.

The aims of the Working Party were two-fold:

1. To consider alternative proposals for the design of machine-readable labels and put forward recommendations to the RTD committee.

2. To ensure that any recommendations have sufficient flexibility to allow for differing needs of Regional Centres.

The latter point is clearly important since the work pattern of RTCs differ and whilst some compromise can be entertained to provide a certain uniformity, it will not be possible for each Centre to operate in the same manner. Also, certain RTCs have specific problems which may be important; for instance, the geography and the population spread in the Region.

An early decision of the Working Party was to follow the American Blood

Commission's recommendations with respect to the details of the bar codes for various products. This will avoid duplication in the numerics of the bar codes which would have occurred if a separate system had been devised for the United Kingdom. The designs for the labels, however, did not always follow the ABC recommendations.

Labels Denoting Donation Number

The first label to be produced was that giving the donation number. The design of those in use currently by five of the six Regions uses the automated grouping equipment. The labels are presented in pads of 150 labels with six labels to each page. Each set of labels comprises four bar-coded labels with the appropriate number above each bar code and two eye-readable numbers only. Thus six labels

Fig 1

0000204	0000204	0000203	0000203
0000204	0000204	0000203	0000203
0000204	0000204	0000203	0000203
0000202	0000202	0000201	0000201
0000202	0000202	0000201	0000201
0000202	0000202	0000201	0000201
0000200	0000200	0000199	0000199
0000200	0000200	0000199	0000199
0000200	0000200	0000199	0000199

are available for attachment to the main pack, transfer pack(s), specimen tubes and donor records.

The need for segregation of new donors from those who had donated previously in the Oxford Region was met by overprinting the pages of labels with a green strip (Fig 2). The advantages of segregating new donors it was considered are two-fold:

1. The specimen tubes from new donors can be separated in the laboratory without tedious checking of numbers and tests, eg for HbsAg, can be carried out before blood grouping.

2. When the computer system proposed in the Oxford Region is completed new donors will be grouped twice and the groups compared before the packs are labelled. Colour coding will allow easy identification of the appropriate tube.

Fig 2

Green ▼   Green ▼

0000210	0000210	0000209	0000209
0000210	0000210	0000209	0000209
0000210	0000210	0000209	0000209
0000208	0000208	0000207	0000207
0000208	0000208	0000207	0000207
0000208	0000208	0000207	0000207
0000206	0000206	0000205	0000205
0000206	0000206	0000205	0000205
0000206	0000206	0000205	0000205

The blocks of six numbers have caused problems on sessions in various Regions. Partly this has been technical in that labels have not separated easily and no doubt this can be resolved. However, the labels must be torn off the sheet sequentially and, particularly with certain left handed persons there is a tendency to tear from left to right. This can lead to the problem of recording one number on the donor record sheet and issuing the donor with a different set of numbers.

The decision initially to have blocks of six sets of numbers to a page was made on economic grounds. However, it has been agreed that in future, sets of donation numbers will be produced in single pads. Two Regions using the labels have now had the blocks of six separated into single sets and an example of the label used in Brentwood for new donors is shown on the right.

Fig 3

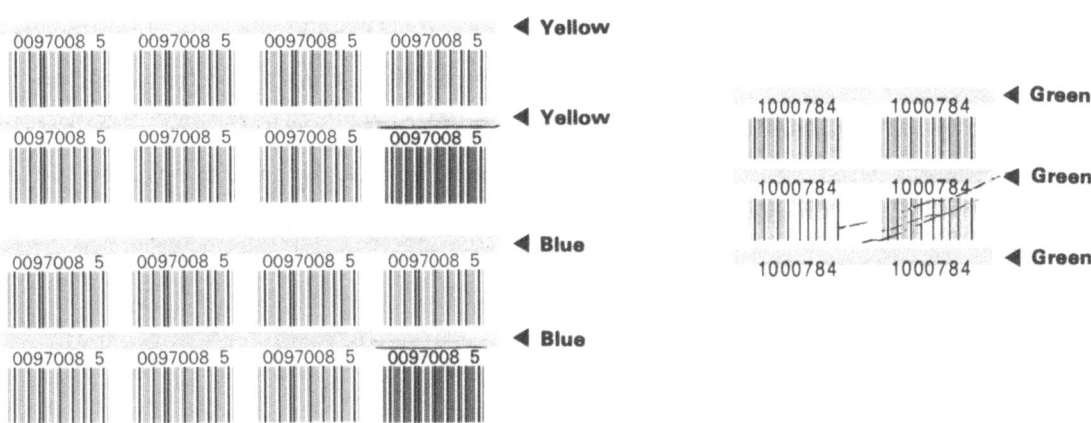

43

It will be noticed that the green bar is placed horizontally through the eye-readable number.

The two sets of labels on the left are those used in the Birmingham Region and obtained from a different manufacturer. Each set comprises eight bar coded labels and the pads are colour coded by a horizontal coloured line to denote the four ABO groups and a green line for new donors. Also, after the eye-readable number, a check digit is included. These sets of labels are presented singly in packs but various defects have been found, eg missing numbers. The latter set of labels are usually removed at the quality control procedure and although the missing numbers are quoted on the top of each pack, the Working Party considers that efforts should be made to avoid such occurrences.

It will have been noted that each donation is identified by 7 digits and, as has been noted above, the labels used in Birmingham also have a check digit. Whilst it is no major problem to read 7 digits with mechanical devices, indeed this is obligatory in the machines in use at present, the manual recording of 7 digits can be a potential source of error. The attention of the Working Party has been drawn to this problem by several hospitals. Moreover, the present labels carry the first number to indicate the Centre of origin. This was inserted so that the origin of blood products could be determined when sent from one Region to another. Since there are 15 Regions, such a policy would lead, eventually, to the first two digits being allocated to identify the RTC. Since 7 digits are required for the grouping machine, this would entail a progression to 8 digits in all and would increase the problems of manual recording both in the RTC and in hospitals. Further consideration however has led to the conclusion that initial digits to identify the RTC are unnecessary providing all blood to hospitals in any one Region is issued from the RTC in that Region. If blood donations or products are transferred directly from on Region to another, they should be transferred from one RTC to that in the receiving Region and not directly from the RTC of one Region to hospitals in another Region. Since each labelled blood pack will have a bar code specifying the Region, it will be possible to record blood issued from another Region prior to re-issue, once computerisation is available. The Working Party has agreed, therefore, that it will recommend that donation numbers will be Regional numbers only and will be restricted to a maximum of 7 digits. Indeed, it is hoped that a reduction from 7 to 6 digits will be a possibility for the future.

RTC Bar Codes

The bar code for the RTC comprises a code for the country, followed by the code
for the RTC which for England and Wales will comprise the DHSS number. The
agreed codes for the countries in the UK are shown in Table I. Each bar code
must comprise 7 digits and, therefore, three digits remain to identify sub-Centres.
The derivation of the bar code for the Oxford RTC is shown in Table I.

Overstick Labels On Blood Packs

Fig 4 illustrates the three positions on the modified label on the main blood
pack which are available for the attachment of informative labels.

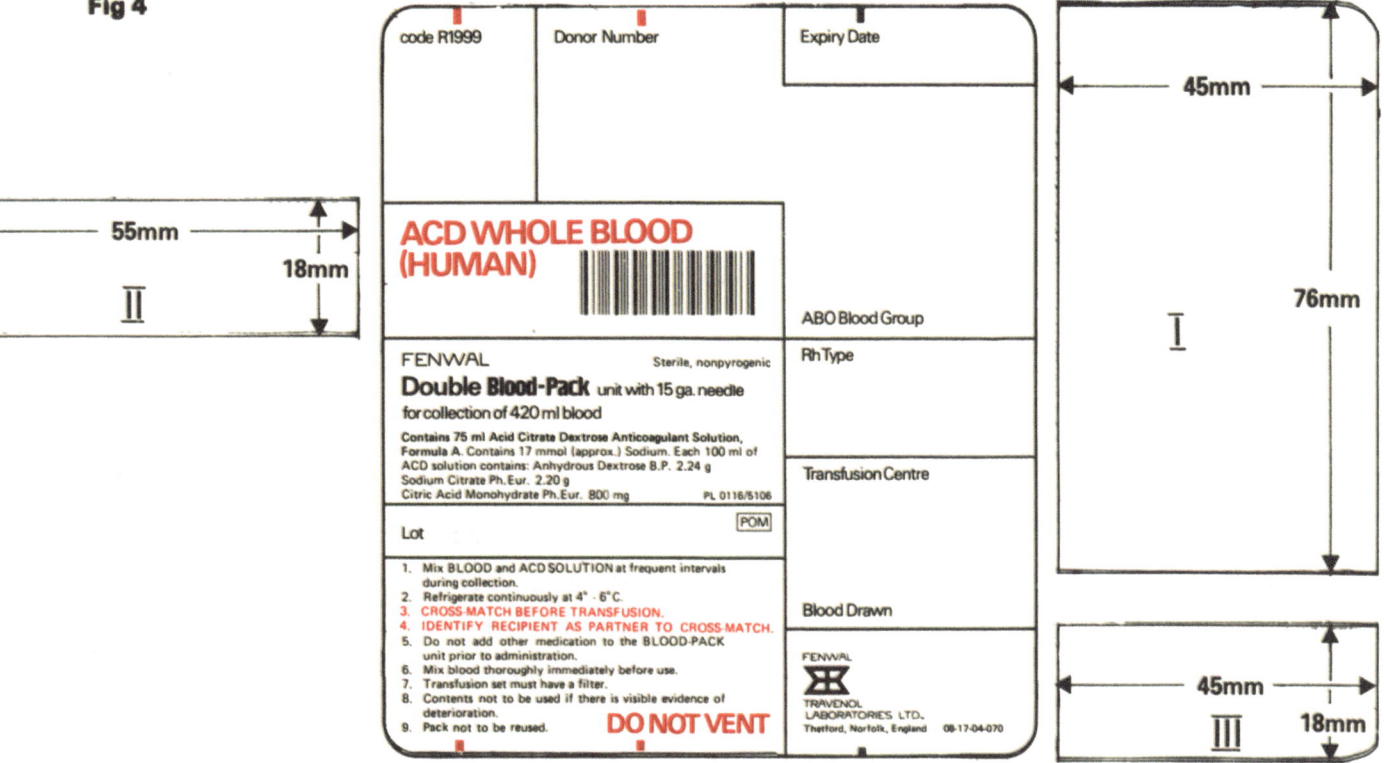

Fig 4

These labels have to conform to a pre-determined size in order not to obliterate
other information on the pack label. The Working Party recommend that labels
which are attached to positions I and II should be uniform and hopefully
acceptable to all Regions so that the advantages of standardisation and economy
can be obtained. Position III however, can be used for labels required locally,
eg to donate CMV-antibody negative, R_1R_1 Kell negative blood etc.

Examples of the ABO and Rh group labels, which are attached at position I are shown in Fig 5. Each label comprises the main label, colour coded appropriately which will peel off the backing paper. Space is available for recording expiry date and date of collection and each label carries the name of the RTC and its appropriate bar code. At the bottom of each label are optional labels denoting the ABO and Rh group since such labels are essential for the procedures in certain RTCs.

Fig 5

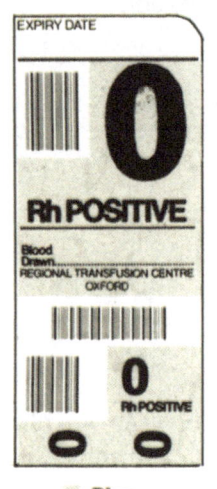 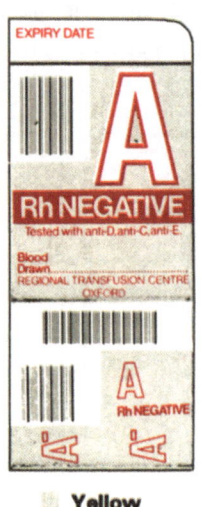 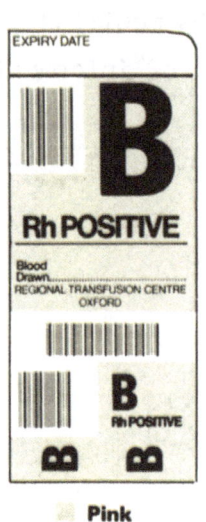

Blue   Yellow   Pink

Fig 6

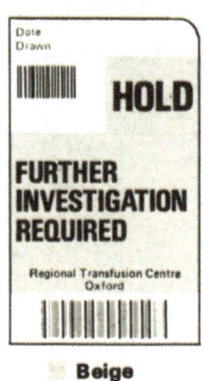 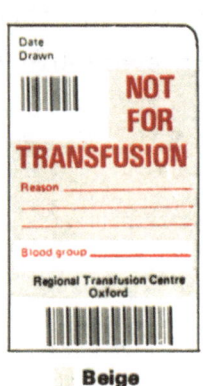 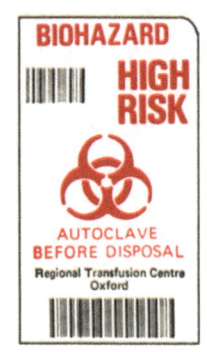

Beige   Beige

Other labels which may be required for position I on the main pack are illustrated in Fig 6. Thus the "HOLD" label is attached to the pack if the blood group is discrepant or in other circumstances where further investigation of the donor's blood is required before issue. If the difficulty is resolved, the appropriate blood group label can be attached over the "HOLD" label. If the blood is found to be unsuitable for issue then a "NOT FOR TRANSFUSION" label will be overstuck. This allows space for giving the reason for unsuitability. At the Brentwood RTC a further label will be used which states "RED CELLS NOT FOR CLINICAL USE, USE FOR PLASMA ONLY". Finally a "BIOHAZARD" label is available which will be used principally when a donation is found to be HbsAg positive.

Labels which can be attached at position II on the main pack are illustrated in Fig 7. Each is descriptive of the product and will cover the designation whole blood. At present five are proposed and comprise: concentrated red cells, plasma reduced blood, saline-washed red cells, thawed and washed red cells which have been stored in the frozen state, and leucocyte-poor blood. Each label bears the bar code appropriate to the product.

Fig 7

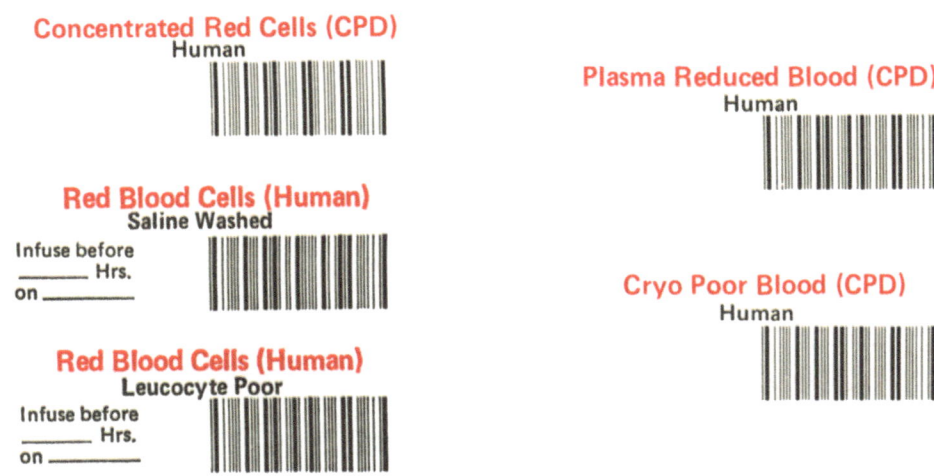

With respect to the satellite pack, there are again three positions for overstick labels (Fig 8). Fortunately positions I and II are the same size as those on the main pack. Position I can be used for the same labels as the main pack, but at position II the label describing the product will usually be different since the product will not consist of a red cell preparation. Examples of product labels are shown in Fig 9 and comprise: platelet concentrates, platelet rich plasma, fresh-frozen plasma and cryoprecipitate.

Fig 8

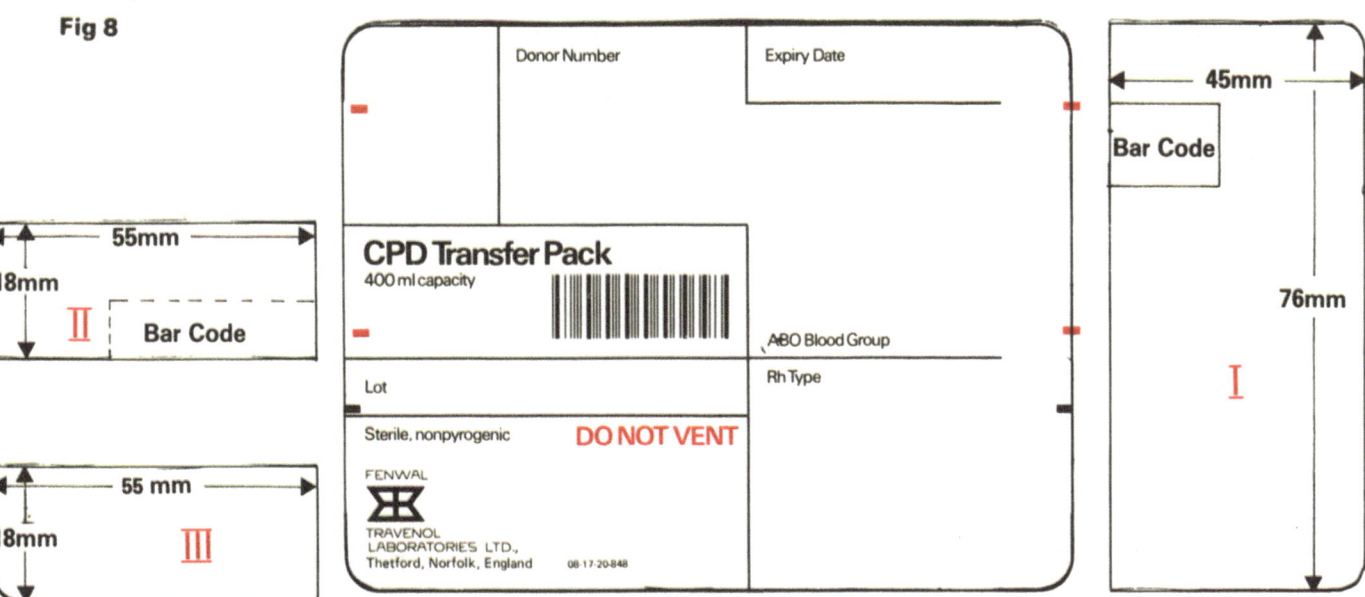

It will be noted by reference to Fig 8 that these labels overstick the bar code on the pack which denotes an empty pack.

Fig 9

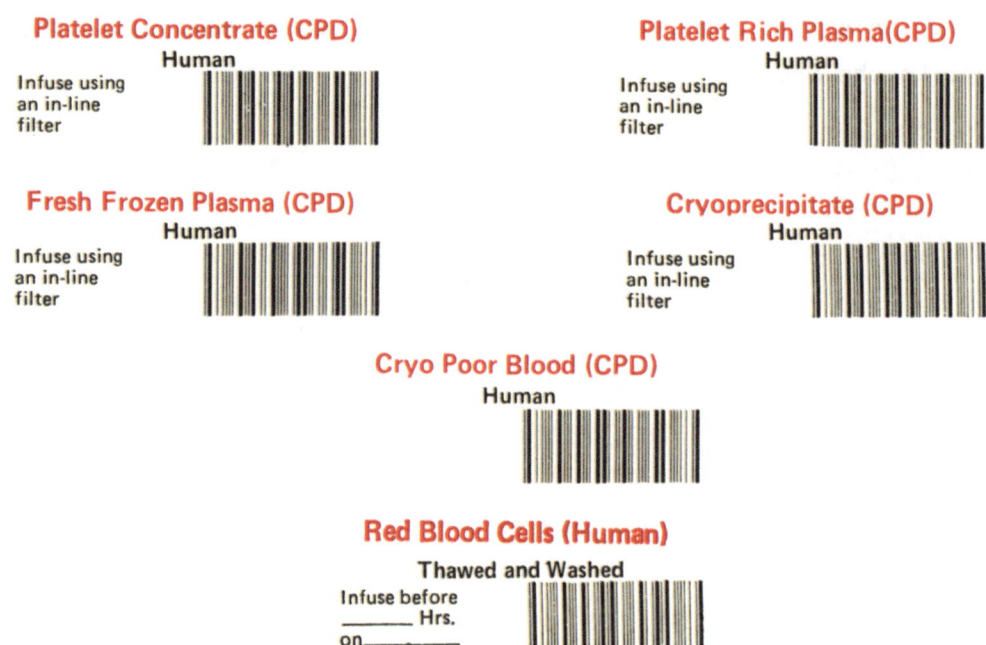

Personal Numbers For Donors

The Working Party has also considered the question of allocation of personal numbers for donors and did give some thought to the question whether this could be done on a National basis which might hold some advantage if donors move from one Region to another. After consideration, however, this suggestion was rejected by the Working Party as impractical for the following reasons:

1.   The donor record card was not being retained in all Regions following the introduction of computer facilities. Indeed these have been dispensed with already in the Birmingham Region. Thus, transfer of donors will vary from Region to Region with the documentation available.

2.   A check digit for numerical input to the computer was required in certain Regions.

3.   With the number of donors enrolled in the NBTS the donor number would have to comprise at least seven digits.

The Working Party will recommend, therefore, that the personal donor number should be allocated Regionally. It is possible, then, to restrict this number to a maximum of six digits.

If a donor transfers from one Region to another, then the Region to which he is transferring will regard him as a new donor. Thus, his existing donor number will be cancelled and he will be given a new number by the Region receiving him/her in a manner similar to any other new donor in that Region.

Allocation Of Numbers To Hospitals

Finally, consideration has been given to the allocation of numbers to hospitals. Relatively little issuing of blood takes place from an RTC in one Region directly to a hospital in another Region, and indeed if the recommendations of this Working Party are observed, this practice will cease. The allocation of numbers to hospitals therefore is a Regional problem and indeed many Regions may wish to follow the example of the Birmingham Region where letter codes are used to identify hospitals.

Conclusion

The report I have given is in some senses a preliminary one. The Working Party has still much to consider. Proposals put forward have yet to be tried out in the field and it is essential that experience is gained in using the labels before the final recommendations are made.

Doubtless in the future, RTCs will require other labels for their use and it may be that they wish to have these with bar codes. It is essential that the bar codes for product labels are agreed internationally. The International Society for Blood Transfusion is the authority approving bar codes and the new ones used in the UK, eg for plasma reduced blood, have been agreed by them. It is hoped that suggestions will be made to the Working Party from RTCs. If agreement can be reached with respect to unformity of the principal labels used in the Service there are obvious economic advantages.

BAR CODE FOR RTC

Comprise:	Code for Country		NW Thames	5
Thus:	England	70	NE Thames	6
	Scotland	71	SE & SW Thames	7/8
	Wales	72	Wessex	9
	N Ireland	73	Oxford	10
			S Western	11
	Code for RTC - DHSS number		W Midlands	12
Thus:	Northern	1	Mersey	13
	Yorkshire	2	N Western	14
	Trent	3	Wales	
	East Anglia	4	RTC Cardiff	15

Code for sub-Centre - (if applicable)

Example: Oxford RTC

7010000

DISCUSSION

Dr BIRD (Birmingham):   Dr Gunson has put over his subject clearly and concisely.

I have two comments.

First, it is true that occasionally because of printing defects the printers of these bar-coded labels leave out one or two numbers so that there are gaps in the sequence. We discovered to our horror, not so long ago, another possible defect. Apparently the printing machine sometimes stammers and turns out two numbers which are exactly the same. This does matter and great care should be taken to see that this possibility is borne in mind.

Secondly, something I was very interested to hear - and Dr Gunson is quite right - and it has to do with inter-regional transfers. It is best that these go from Centre to Centre. I feel rather bad about this now. It is only the other day that a patient was transferred from one of the Birmingham hospitals to Hammersmith, and they would not accept this patient unless he was accompanied by eight units of Group B positive blood because it was alleged that they could not get any from the appropriate transfusion centre. I authorised the despatch of these eight units but I now see that I should not have done that. I should have routed them through the appropriate Blood Transfusion Centre. I do not know if the hospital at Hammersmith would have liked that particularly, but I shall take note of this for the future.

Dr WILKINSON (Dublin):   What is the difference between plasma reduced blood and concentrated red cells?

Dr GUNSON: Plasma-reduced blood in this context has between 180-200 ml plasma removed from whole blood which results in a packed cell volume of between 60 and 65%. Concentrated red cells usually have a packed cell volume in excess of 70%. Over the years I have found that in order to make red preparations more acceptable to clinicians, the packed cell volume has to be kept down to prevent slowing of the transfusion. Anaesthetists and surgeons in operative situations cannot accept a slow drip rate and this leads them to demand whole blood or to dilute the red cell preparation with plasma protein fraction.

Dr IBBOTSON: I think there is a difference in terminology. We use the term 'concentrated red cells' when we have the haemotocrit at 70 which is quite acceptable and presents no problems to the clinicians. Nor does the terminology put them off using red cell concentrates.

Dr CASH: There is indeed a difference in terminology and we will need first and foremost to agree on the terms to be used and the specifications for each type of blood product so defined.

Dr GUNSON: Perhaps the difference in terminology is due to the fact that the term 'plasma reduced blood' was suggested by the World Health Organisation in their report on 'Proposed Requirements for the Production and Quality Control of Human Blood Products and Related Substances', whereas the definition of concentrated red cells given in the British Pharmacopeia allows a much wider interpretation.

Dr CASH: Once these features have been agreed their implementation will have a considerable impact on production schedules at Regional Centres.

Dr GUNSON: I think I should point out that the labels shown are advisory and do not have to be used by anyone. If the procedure in a particular Regional Transfusion Centre is such that it is not considered that plasma reduced blood fits the description of the red cell product, then there is an alternative label for concentrated red cells.

Prof STRATTON: In passing, in a revealing few words, Dr Gunson said that they like to know the new donors because they put them through the machine twice. Does this mean that his system is of a very dubious accuracy?

Dr GUNSON: Not necessarily. We have been using the Groupamatic system for a relatively short time and we have not yet assessed its full potential. Dr Wagstaff has used it for longer and may have more confidence in grouping his new donors once only. However any grouping can result in error, be it frequent or infrequent. With a donor whose group is known it is possible to compare the group following a given donation with the stated group of the donor found on a previous occasion.

In our Region we considered it was prudent to have a check following the grouping of a new donor and the only way was to carry it out twice. With the capacity of this machine of 360 groups an hour, no difficulty is posed in carrying out this procedure within a normal working day.

Prof STRATTON: So Dr Gunson is saying that the manual method is the most reliable method of doing groups.

Dr GUNSON: No, I would not necessarily go as far as that. I think that errors can occur in manual methods as well as in automated methods. When one is grouping packs to issue for transfusion one should be as prudent as one may.

Our experience over the past few months with this particular machine is that it is extremely reliable. So far we have found no discrepancies in the duplicate groups of our new donors. But I would hesitate not to do it all the same.

Dr SMITH (Southampton):   I understand from a recent visit to the Oxford Centre that new donors are distinguished from old so that an Au antigen test can be done before the blood groups are determined by machine.

All our new donors at Southampton are grouped manually as well as by machine, but we have a Technicon 15 channel machine, not one of the newer machines with laser identification of samples by bar coding.

Dr WAGSTAFF (Sheffield): To answer Prof Stratton's question - indirectly. We have used the machine for two and a half years now. If one accepts that a rejected group is a correct decision of the machine drawing attention to something wrong, then in $2\frac{1}{2}$ years this has missed one group which we knew from previous occasions was an Ax with anti-A which acted against both A_1 and A_2 cells. That has been the only fallacy in $2\frac{1}{2}$ years.

Prof STRATTON: But running it twice would not have helped, would it?

Dr WAGSTAFF: No.

Dr BIRD: Firstly, one cannot blame Dr Wagstaff's machine for making that particular mistake. That was what it had to find on the evidence before it.

If one looks closely at everything that has been written about Ax, one will find that the antibody that is present in the serum is not really an anti-A1, it is an anti-A. I am therefore not surprised that when it is strong it will agglutinate both A-1 and A-2 cells.

This is not really relevant to our discussions but it refers to Dr Wagstaff's comment.

Dr NAPIER: We received the starting digit of 6, and on inspection of the samples it seemed to me that 6's, 9's, 0's and 8's can all be read either way up - and there are a certain number of numbers that can be read either way, upside down or the correct way. That seems to be important for the single strips of numbers - but obviously not when there is an integral bar code.

Has Dr Gunson found this to be the case in practice?

Dr JENKINS: The Working Party looked at this and it is true. The eye-readable numbers can be turned upside down and one can read an intelligent number. We went through a phase of using the first character to identify the centre and this safeguarded us up to a point. Brentwood was always 1 and we always read 1-something and knew that we had it the right way up.

Now that we are going away from centre identification and we may start with zeros, we shall have to consider it again. It may be necessary to put a line to indicate which way up the label has to be read. We shall be discussing this at the Working Party.

PROPOSAL FOR THE INTRODUCTION OF BAR CODED LABELS
AND DATA PROCESSING IN REGIONAL TRANSFUSION CENTRES IN UK
Mr G Williams (Regional Transfusion Centre, Brentwood)

I should like to discuss a proposed data processing system to utilise bar coded
labels, with these labels being the central theme of the system. This is not an
established system yet but a proposal, although one part of the system is due
to be in operation by the end of June 1979.

Many of the functions in transfusion centres involve much manual transcription,
and each transcription is subject to error. It is generally agreed that the use
of machine readable labels provides an ideal solution to the problem; the labels
used in this application are CODABAR. The use of such labels also solves the
problem of data input to a data processing system. Data must be entered as
typed entries, on punched cards or using bar-coded labels. The problems of
typed entries are obvious and are eliminated using bar code. The following
Proposal highlights four areas where bar-code can be applied.

SESSIONS	Check donor details Assign unit number Enter donation details
LABORATORY	Add test results Check previous results
SORT	Check labelling Add over-stick labels
ISSUE	Log issues/returns

Beginning at sessions, light pens can be used to check donor details by reading
a bar-coded donor number from a donor identity card. Donor information can be
displayed at a VDU screen for checking. By wanding the donor number in this way,
the donor's attendance is automatically registered. Light pens can also be used
in assigning unit numbers, wanding first the donor number and then immediately
wanding the unit number. This provides the association of donor identity with
unit identity right from the time of the session where the unit is taken. Finally
donation details can be recorded using light pens to wand appropriate coded
remarks from a bar-code menu, thus making the task of recording such details much
easier than typing into a terminal.

The second application is found in the laboratory testing of samples. Here this
proposal deals with testing by Groupamatic equipment, but could equally apply
to Technicon equipment which also uses a laser reader to interpret bar-coded
sample numbers. The laser reader scans the sample number on the pilot tube and
matches the number with the results obtained for the sample. The computer then
checks any previous results and warns of any anomaly. The third application is in
the sorting and labelling of blood, and it is here that the greatest advantage
of using bar-code really becomes apparent. Two systems may operate: either packs
arrive in the centre with no group label, in which case they have to be both
labelled and checked, or the packs arrive with group labels already attached and
these have only to be checked. Either system may be used with equal security
using bar-coded labels.

The fourth application to be considered is in the issue department. Here,
inventory control is achieved by logging issues and returns of blood by wanding
labels with light pens. The destination of units may be recorded similarly and
thus blood can be traced very rapidly if necessary.

The following sections deal with each application in greater detail.

1.   Sessions

It is planned to take to sessions a portable micro-computer with a light pen.
Also taken will be floppy discs containing donor details of the entire panel plus
details of all the donors called to a particular session. By wanding the donor
number, the details are found on the disc file by the computer and displayed.
Only if the donor does not belong to the panel will the details not be available,
and the donor will be treated as a new donor. The use of portable micro-computers
is necessary since many session sites lack telephone facilities and therefore an
on-line link to the central computer is impossible.

After checking the donor details, the haemoglobin test is performed. The result
is recorded by wanding a bar-code from a menu card.

SESSION REMARKS

PRE-DONATION		POST-DONATION	
Hb OK Donation Taken	‖‖‖‖‖‖‖‖	1	‖‖‖‖‖‖‖‖
Low Hb Sample Taken	‖‖‖‖‖‖‖‖	2	‖‖‖‖‖‖‖‖
Low Hb No Sample	‖‖‖‖‖‖‖‖	3	‖‖‖‖‖‖‖‖
Reject	‖‖‖‖‖‖‖‖	4	‖‖‖‖‖‖‖‖
		5	‖‖‖‖‖‖‖‖

Session Menu Card

If the haemoglobin is acceptable a unit number is attached to the pack and wanded.
Figures 3 and 4 show primary and secondary pack labels with and without unit
numbers attached.

Identical unit numbers are also attached to three pilot tubes and to a registration
document, which may be a 101 card or some other document. After the donation,
various comments may be entered by wanding, from a menu card, the appropriate
coded remark. If the donor's haemoglobin is low, this will also be recorded with
a light pen. A sample number will be attached to a sample tube and a sample taken
for follow-up testing. This sample number can also be bar-coded since the
haematology results will also be stored by the main computer and the number can
be entered by wanding.

Once the session is ended, the floppy discs are returned to the centre where
their records are transferred to the main system.

2.   Laboratories

Samples are tested for ABO and Rh groups using Groupamatic equipment. This
provides results correlated with sample identification. At the end of each batch,
the results are transferred to the main computer which checks previous results
against current data and warns of any discrepancy or anomaly. Entry of manual
results has to be approached differently. At the present time there is no plan

57

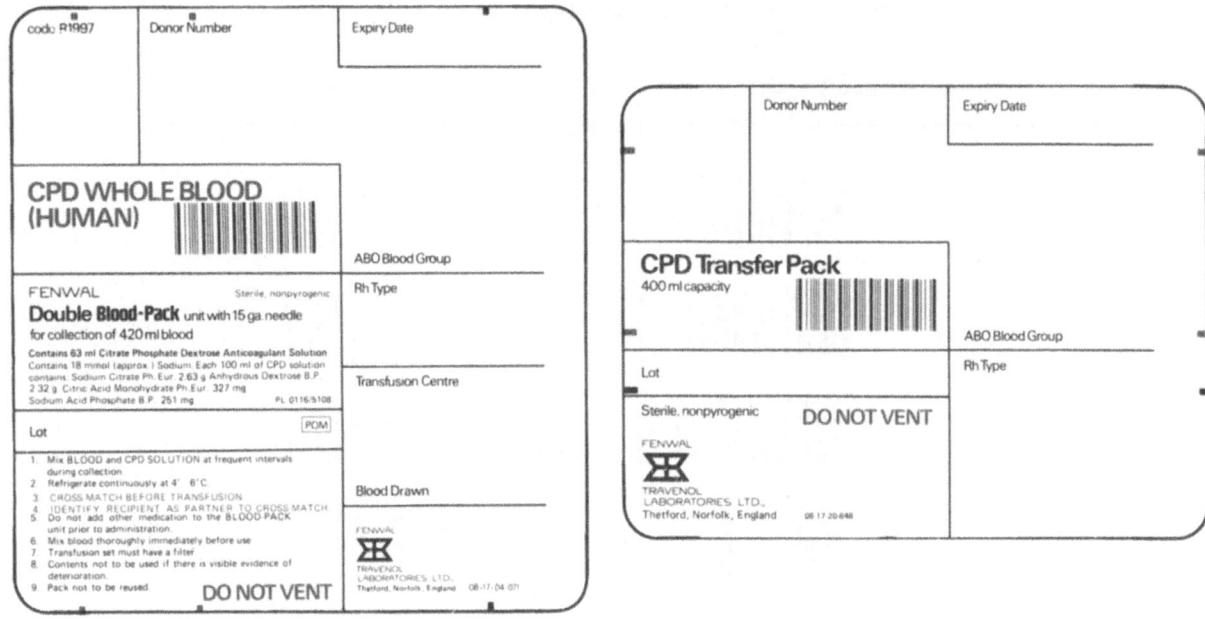

Fig 3 Primary and secondary packs without unit numbers

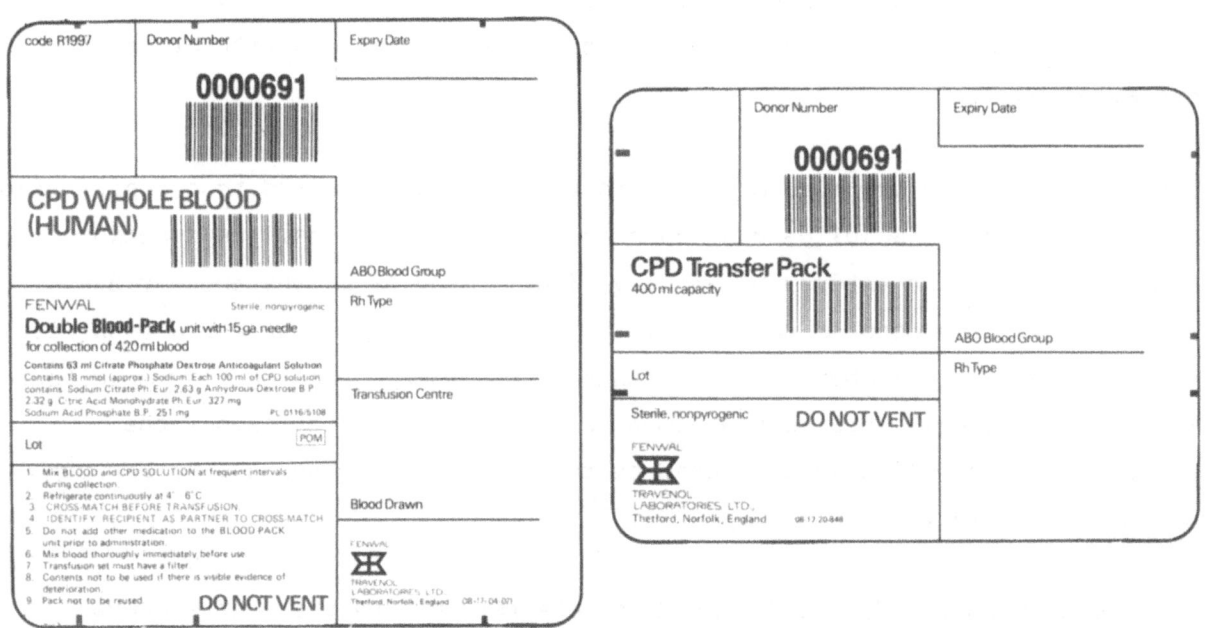

Fig 4 Pack labels with unit numbers attached

to use bar-code to enter manual test results. However, bar-code is used in the New York Blood Centre for this function, and it is an area requiring further investigation. The present proposal is to enter manual results at keyboards, and this is the only area where keyboard entry will be required to any extent. This is as a result of using bar coded menu cards or labels for all other data entry including calling programmes at a terminal.

3.   Blood sort

This description assumes that blood packs are received without group labels and staff sorting blood will get the packs with a unit number only. This number will be wanded with a light pen resulting in a display of the group together with any other relevant details and sorting information. Depending on the sort fate assigned to a unit in the laboratory, several possible situations may arise:

a.   The results are in order, and a correct blood group is displayed. In this instance, the correct group label (fig 5) is attached to the pack and the unit number and group code wanded in one sweep of the pen.

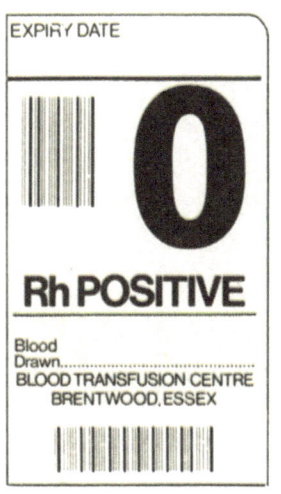
Blue

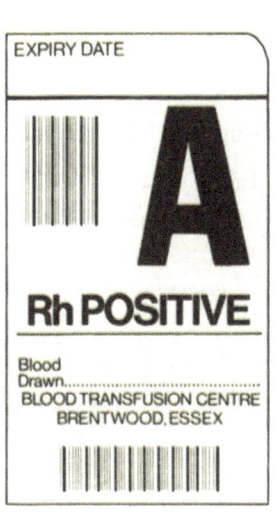
Yellow

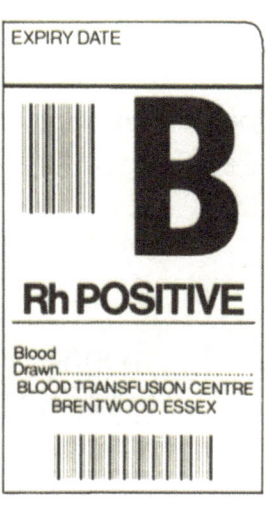
Pink

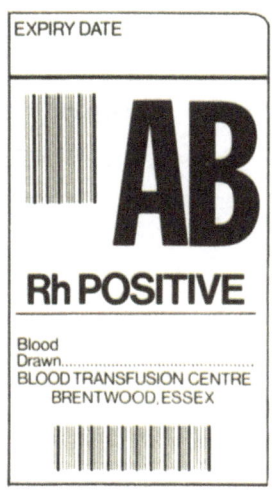

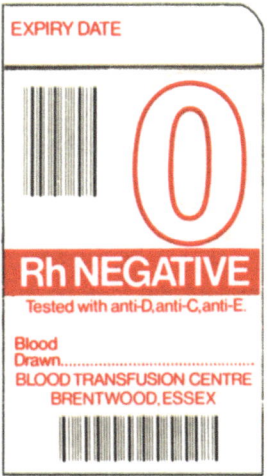

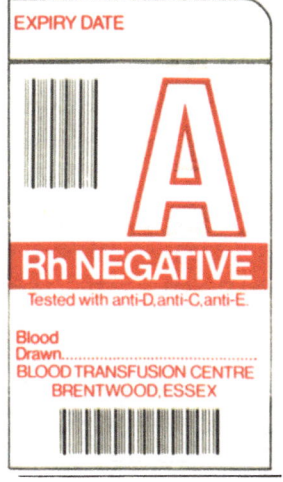

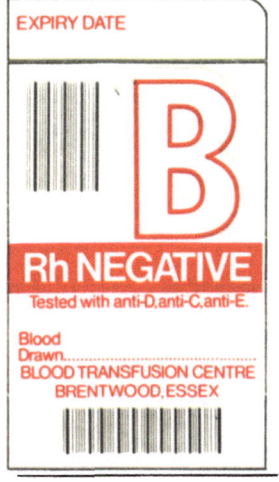

Fig 5   Blood group labels

The number label ends with a d-pause code and the group code begins with d-pause. If the unit number is wanded alone, the d-pause is replaced by the pen with a stop code to indicate the end of the message. This happens after a given time interval lasting several milliseconds. If, however a group code follows immediately after the number, the d-pause at the start of this code cancels that at the end of the number and the number and group code are read as one message. Since the computer will expect a complete message it will reject anything less. The computer then checks that the label is the correct one. Once again, an incorrect label will be rejected. Since the correct label must follow the number label immediately, it is impossible to wand a unit number from one pack with a group label from another. It is therefore impossible to label a pack incorrectly since the computer will not allow the sort to proceed until a correctly labelled pack is rewanded.

b. There may be some reason not to release a unit for issue. For example, there may be an antibody present. In this case, a HOLD label would be attached to the pack (fig 6).

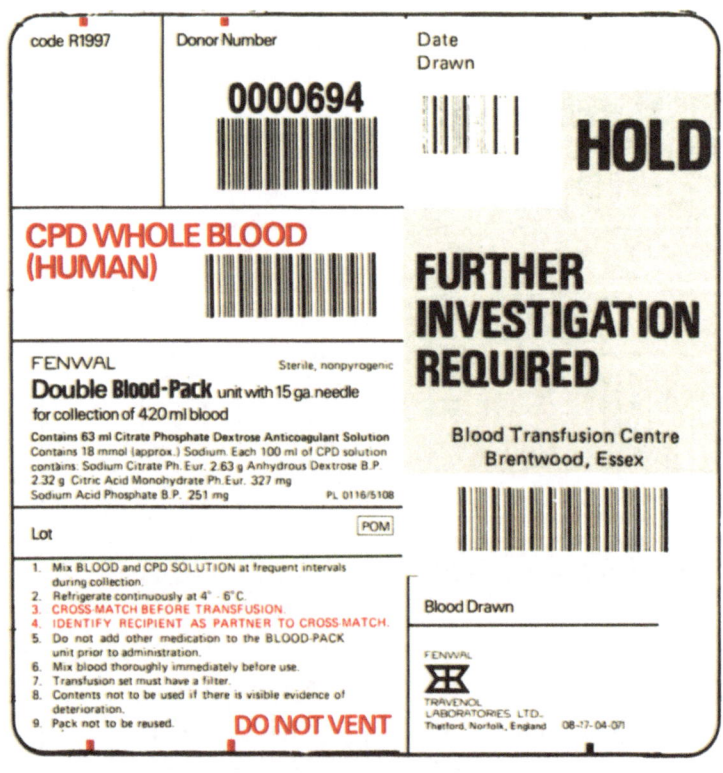

Fig 6 Hold   ▓ **Beige**

The pack is rewanded and the same checking takes place
except that the computer now expects a HOLD label code.
A HOLD label may also be attached by the sort team, even
in the absence of an instruction from the computer to do
so. This is sometimes necessary if the pack is underweight
or faulty in some way. All held packs are subsequently
sorted by a senior technician who decides its fate.

c.   A unit may be totally unfit for issue. In this case a NOT
      FOR TRANSFUSION label is used (fig 7).

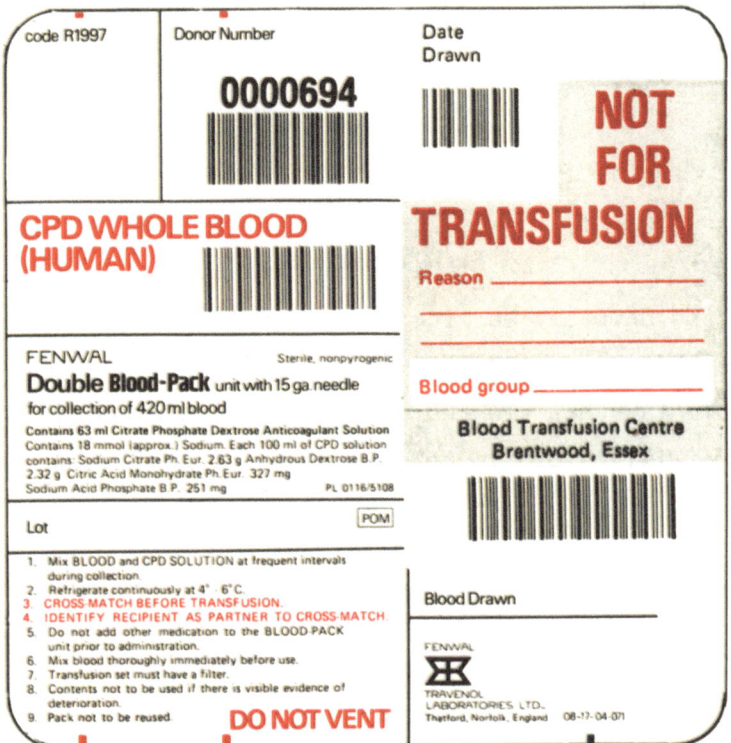

Fig 7 Not for Transfusion   Beige

When rewanded, the computer is informed that the unit is to be
removed from the inventory.

d.   If a unit is found to be hepatitis positive it must obviously
      be discarded and incinerated. A BIOHAZARD label (fig 8) is
      used to inform the computer that correct action will be taken
      and to inform staff handling the unit of its danger.

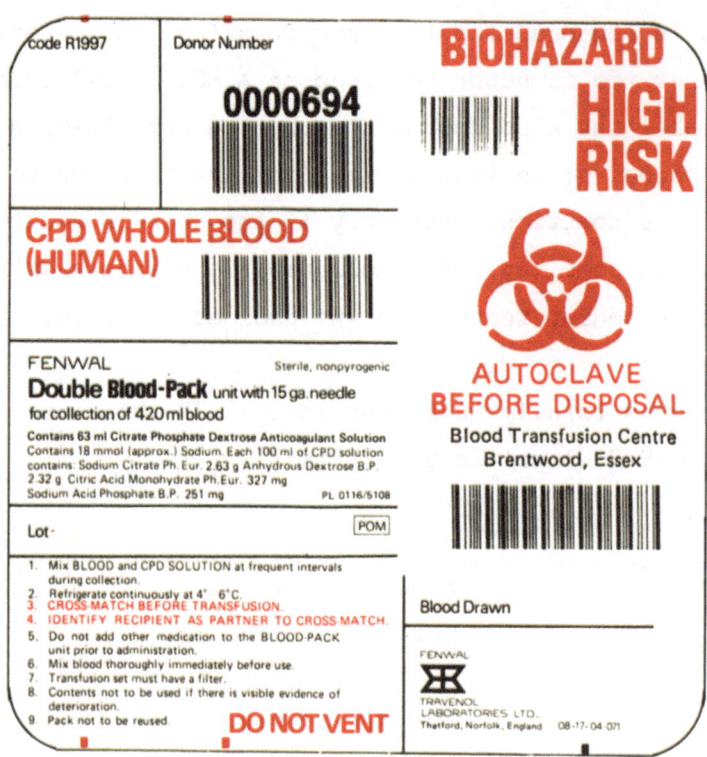

Fig 8 Biohazard

e. Finally, the unit may be from a donor with a history of malaria. For these units, a PLASMA USE ONLY label is used. This indicates to the computer that the red cells are to be discarded but that the plasma will remain in the inventory (see fig 9).

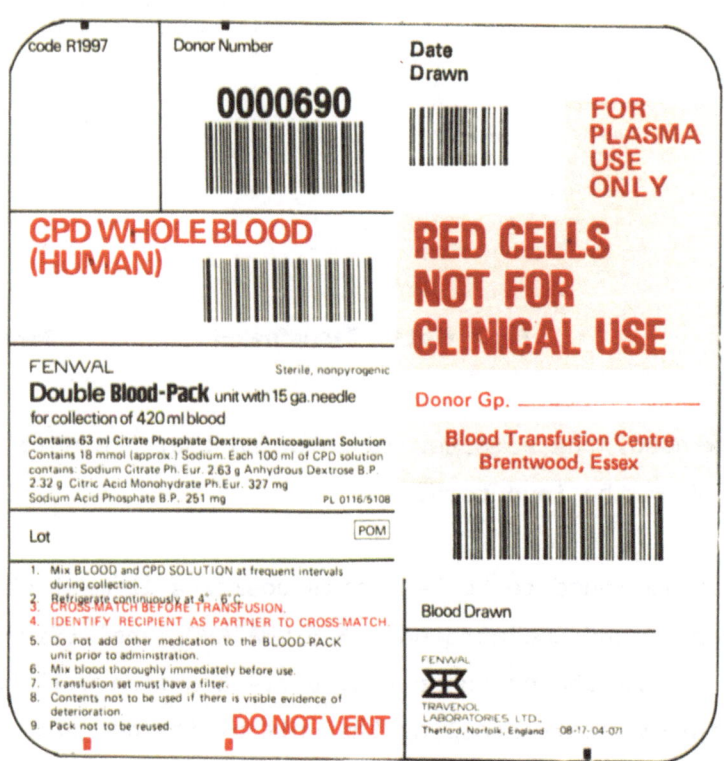

Fig 9 Plasma use only　　　　　　　Beige

The above procedures described for laboratory and sorting procedures are being implemented at Brentwood using micro-computer equipment, and are due to be operational at the end of June 1979.

4. Issue

Having been labelled and passed for issue, the units arrive in the issue department. Some will have been fractionated and have various product labels attached (figs 10-12).

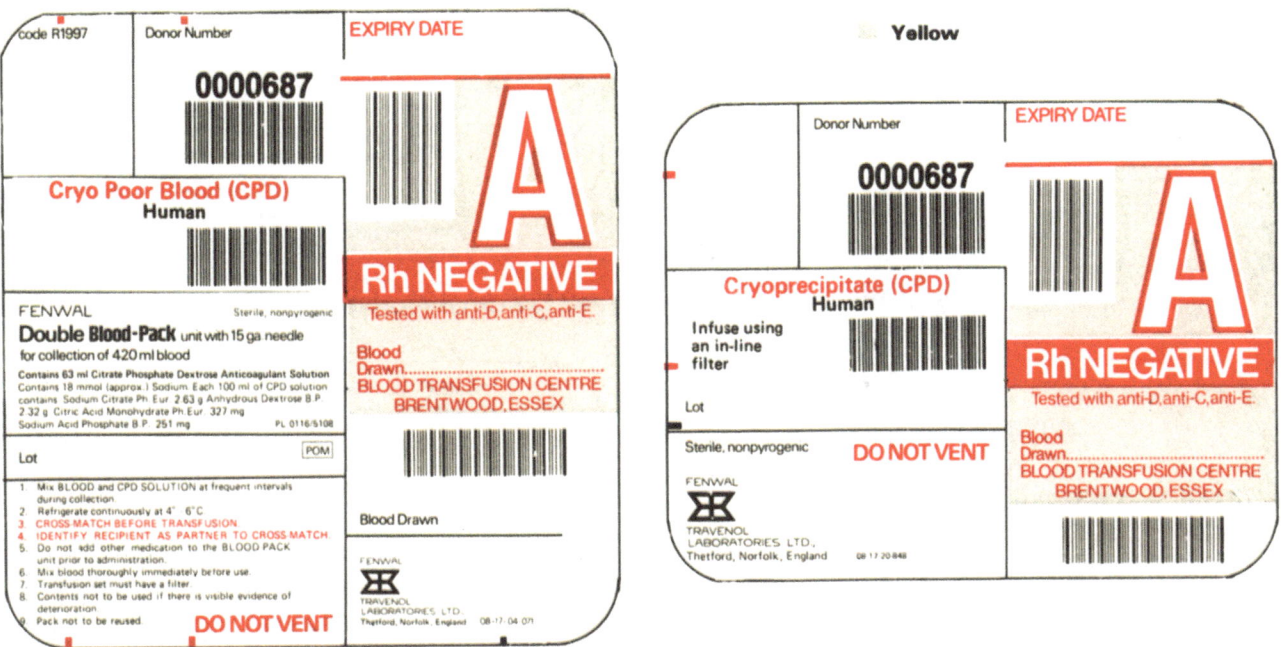

Fig 10 Cryo-Poor Blood and Cryoprecipitate

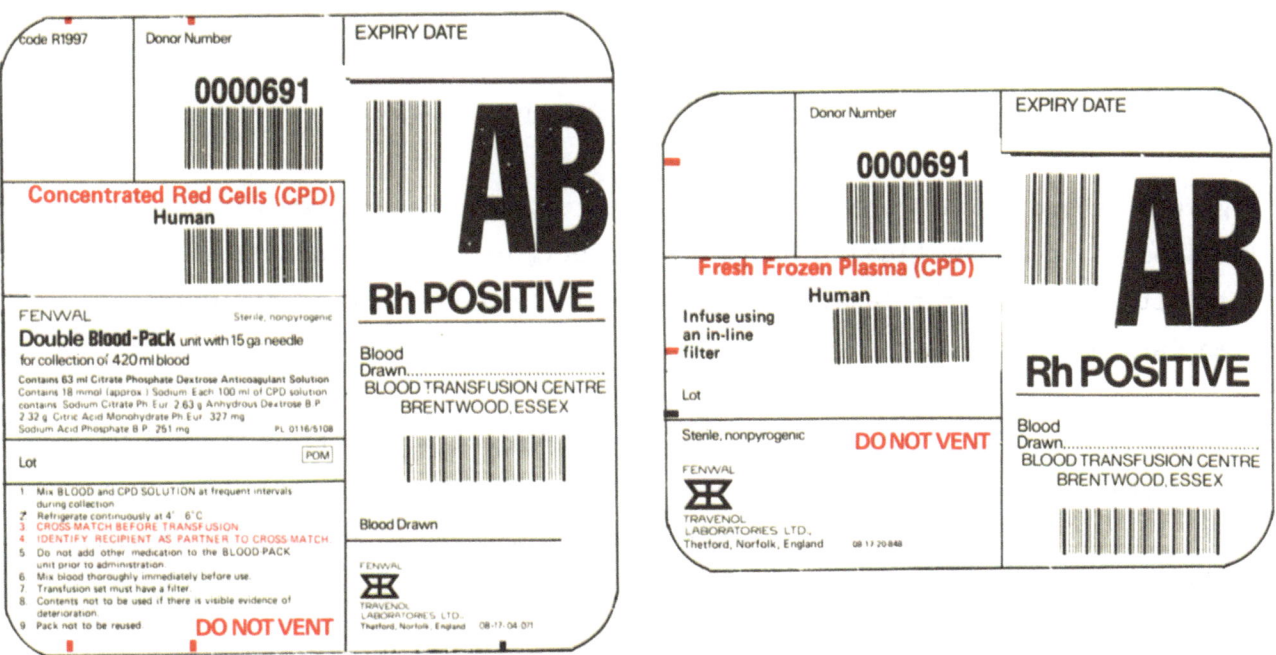

Fig 11 Concentrated Red Cells and Fresh Frozen Plasma

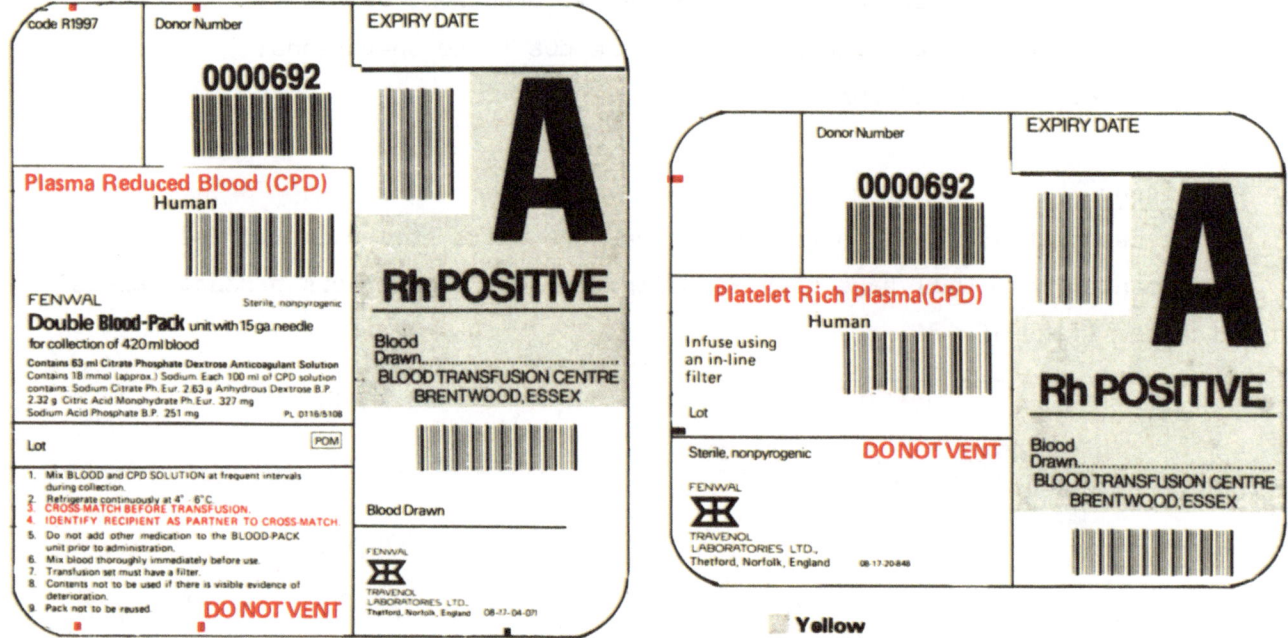

Fig 12 Plasma Reduced Blood and Platelet Rich Plasma

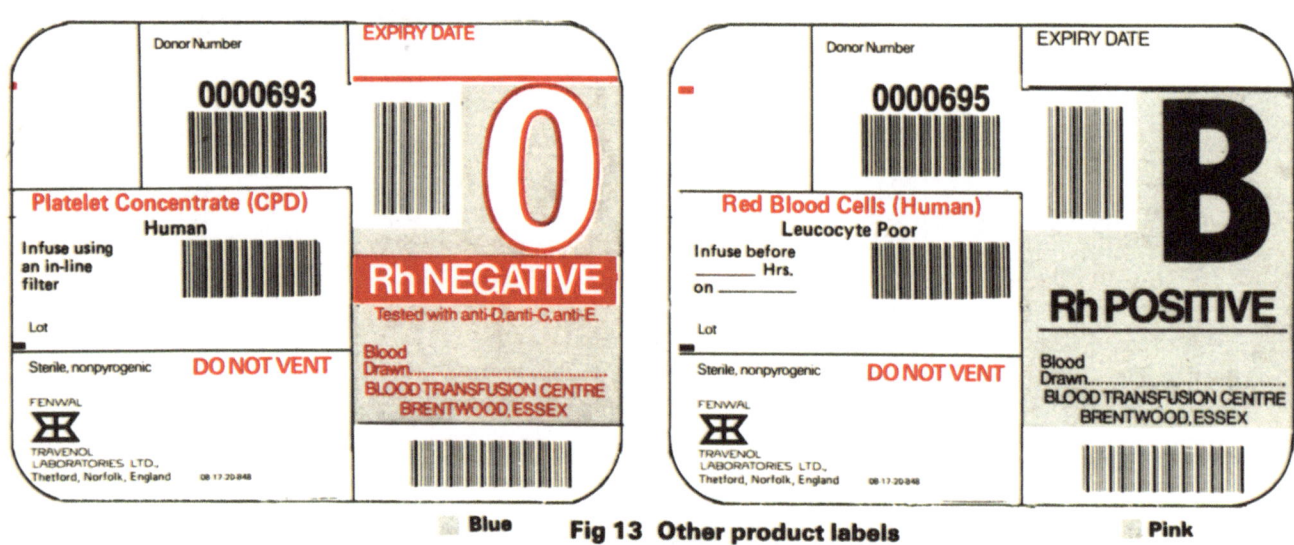

Fig 13 Other product labels

Figure 10 shows a primary pack which has had cryoprecipitate removed and so is labelled as cryo-poor blood in place of the original Whole Blood label. The satellite pack has been labelled as cryoprecipitate in place of the original Transfer pack label.

Figures 11 and 12 similarly show Concentrated Red Cells with Fresh Frozen Plasma and Plasma Reduced Blood with Platelet Rich Plasma. Other product labels are shown in figure 13. All the product labels are bar-coded to allow for inventory control.

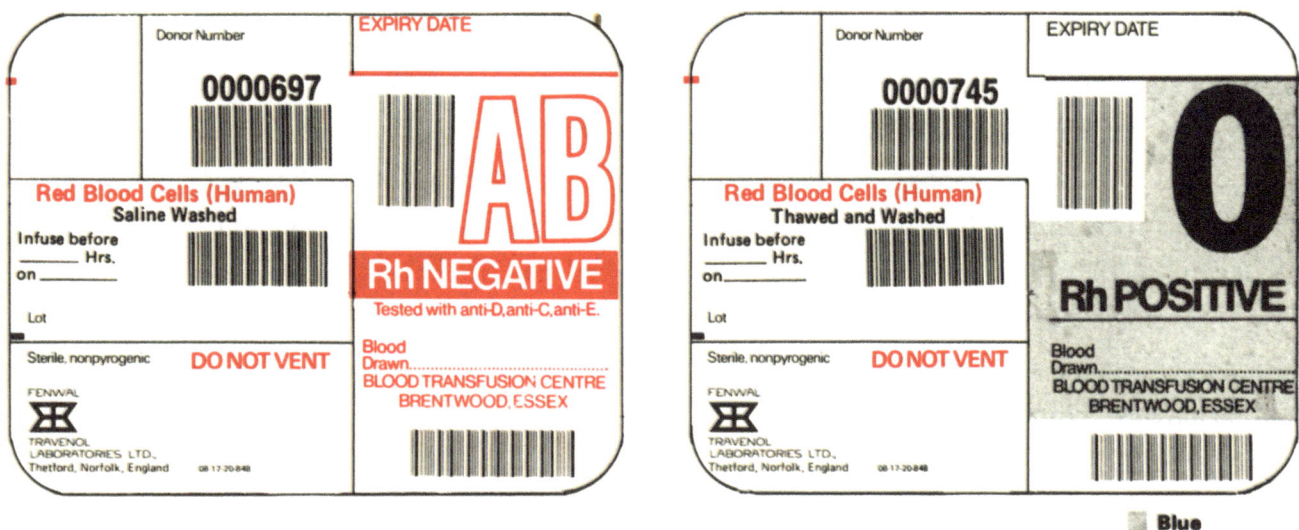

Fig 13 Other product labels

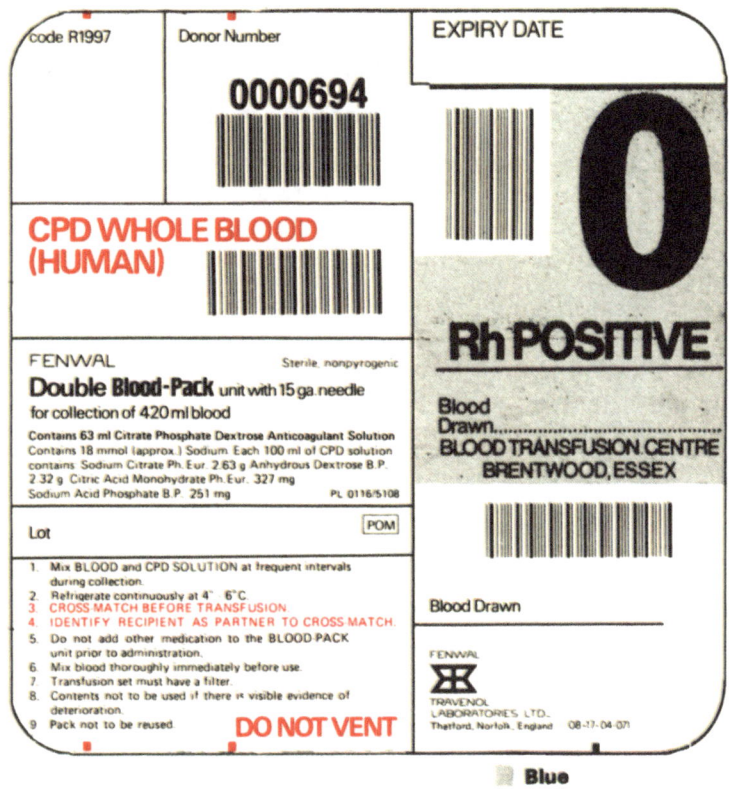

Fig 14 Fully labelled unit

When the pack arrives in the issue department it will have been labelled with a
unit number, a group label and a product label (see fig 14).

When the pack is issued the issue clerk will wand the unit number with a light pen. The group label may also be wanded as an extra check, but by the time it has reached sort the blood group information is already available to the computer; the group of the unit is already on file so there is no need to wand it, but it may be desirable to do so as an extra security check. The product code will also be wanded to indicate which type of product is being issued. If the unit originated in another region, the centre identification will be wanded. This is necessary since there may be two identical unit numbers in different centres. The combination of unit number and centre identity is, however, unique. Finally the clerk will wand the hospital code from a menu card. The unit's destination is thereby recorded and will enable swift tracing if required.

When logging returns of blood, the same procedure applies. The provision of hospital usage statistics thus becomes automatic.

This has been a brief discussion of the proposals for a data processing system intended to utilize bar-coded labels for management of donor records, laboratory results, blood labelling and blood inventory control. Ultimately the use of such labels must spread into hospitals where patient identity can then be matched with unit identity to provide a totally secure method of identification. This will greatly reduce the risks of transfusion that are associated with clerical error.

DISCUSSION

Dr BRODHEIM: One comment. I noticed that the procedure for hold was to assign a unit number prior to medical screening and then to cancel it if the donor is deferred in the medical screening. I believe that there may be some risk in that procedure and I should like to suggest an alternative for consideration - one that we are planning to use. Two sequences of numbers would be assigned to each blood collection site, one for donors who are accepted and the second for donors who are deferred. No assignment would be made until after medical screening, in which case there is no possibility of a mix-up.

In Mr Williams's procedure, if, for any reason, the withdrawal of that number is skipped, the outcome will be duplicate donors for the same number.

Mr WILLIAMS: That is right, yes. One of the problems at the session is an organisational problem. It is very difficult to plan how we would arrange for a donor identity to be married with unit number. It may well be that we have to alter session procedures to accommodate that. It is obviously something that will need a lot more thought given to it.

Dr JENKINS: The fact is that we do the labelling and then pass the donor on for further assessment, by a doctor, so the wrong number may be put on to start with.

Dr CASH: At the point of the sort, when the unit number would be wanded, and then the group checked, and if it was not right the computer would say: Stop, flash lights, and so on, and then one would put on the correct label, wand again, and proceed - could some evil person take a label, not put it physically on to the dontion, but line it up with the unit number, wand through, and then get proceed from the computer?

Mr WILLIAMS: Without sticking it on to the pack?

Dr CASH: Right.

I take that point on because at the point of issue the unit number would be wanded, but not the group as well unless there were special security reasons.

Is it an important point?

Mr WILLIAMS: It might be one reason why we should check it again at issue. Dr Cash could be right. In any system we devise using bar codes there will be some way round it if someone intends to be felonious.

Dr JENKINS: I think it is a good point.

Dr CASH: We have had one episode - not to do with bar codes.

Quarter to five at nights seems to produce weariness and a desire to go home.

IMPLICATIONS FOR HOSPITAL TRANSFUSION DEPARTMENTS

Mr R Fewell (London Hospital)

Mr FEWELL: The computer system at the London Hospital is clinically based.
It is not a laboratory computer. The laboratory is part of the overall system.
It has a clinial connotation and my remarks will have our own system very much
in mind. Various hospitals have various facilities but most are dedicated systems
within the laboratory. At The London we feel - given the patients and the money -
that if we are able to do so we should offer a complete system from donor to
recipient. There is no doubt that the recipient is the most important person in
the chain, and there is no doubt, too, that bar coding will bring a new dimension
to the hospital. Doubtless it will have its problems, but it has considerable
advantages, not least the cutting out of errors in patient identification. Too
many of the mishaps in transfusion have clerical error as the basis.

We feel, too, that it could more readily and conveniently allow monitoring of
specific plasma fraction treatment for purely clinical advantage. With an
on-line system clincially based, it should allow the medical and/or nursing staff
to know when blood is available, whether it has been used and how much is still
available for any one patient from a specific request.

By interfacing from the London with Brentwood, it should be possible to allow
the blood transfusion director or his medical staff access to clinical details
of the patient - a point which might be of interest to the transfusion service.

The system as we see it would be for units of blood or fractionation products
to be issued from the blood transfusion centre according to agreed stock levels.
By agreed stock levels I mean that the transfusion centre - we assume - would
work out and agree with us what would be an agreed stock to hold.

How would this be allocated to the hospital? The stock issue could be wanded out
at the centre and sent to the hospital with an issue checklist, or, we hope, more
appropriately, a list printed out in the hospital and the units checked in
when they arrive. Delivery could be wanded in locally in the London and a printout obtained locally. Whichever method is used, blood would be put into the
stock refrigerator.

I have talked about printouts and checklists. I really believe that this is
something on which the hospital, in liaison with the tranfusion centres, must
insist if we are to have anything like an on line system. It has been my
experience with the pathology computer services at the London that manual input
always carries an error rate, and if large volumes of work have to be handled
then tracing errors can be very time-consuming. Given a printout it is easier to
track down any mistakes, and we would hope to have both a VDU and a local
printer in the blood transfusion laboratory.

From then on as the blood is put into the cross match stream, it would be wanded
out of stock as it is put up for crossmatch, so that the blood transfusion centre
would at all times know the stock position in our particular hospital. It would
also be valuable for the centre to know what the stock position is should it wish
to transfer stock to another hospital or location, thereby saving transport. We
think that the saving in time could be enormous.

It is essential for the laboratory to always be up to date in its stock control.
It is no good postulating these things unless the staff actually carry out,
religiously, the function of in and out wanding, as otherwise the whole system
falls apart.

Having made those few remarks, I am really skirting round the problem. All
that is fairly easy. The nitty-gritty in all this is how to label the patient
and as far as we are concerned, in our neck of the woods it is this problem which
poses most difficulty. I was very interested to hear Dr Brodheim say that in
New York they have started to set up an experimental model to investigate this.
We are thinking of doing the same.

Before I say more about that, perhaps I might show one or two illustrations of
our system to show what it can offer not only to other disciplines in pathology
but to the blood transfusion and blood group serology service as well. The system
supplies requesting, data processing and reporting. It is a total system, and like
all total systems it is pretty inconvenient on a Sunday afternoon.

Nevertheless this is a model of the services which are offered. A lot of it would

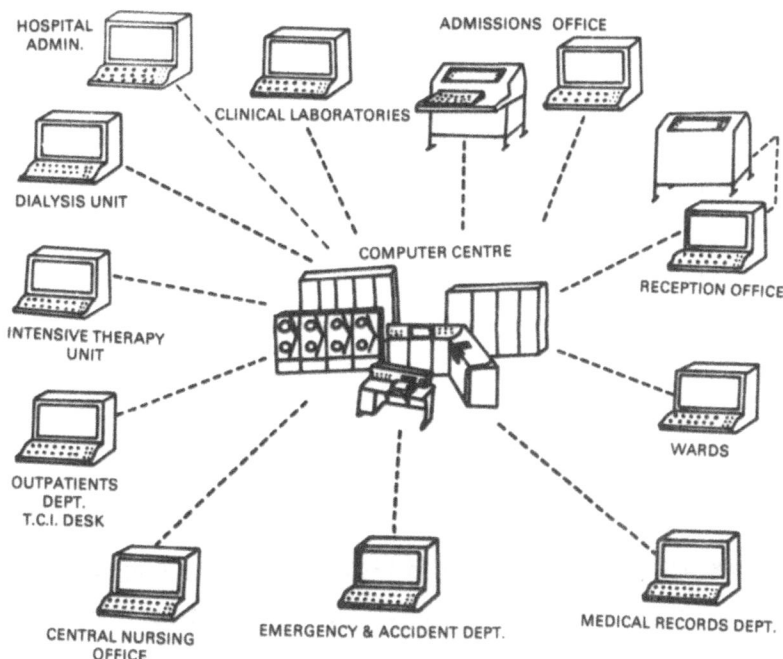

just be of passing interest to this audience but it does show the complete package
including the clinical laboratories. All the departments are there, including
the admissions office which is an important part of our system because if a
hospital is to have an on-line system for blood transfusion work, or for any other
work, then it really must have a master index. The next illustration is a mock
up of the haemotology system as it stands at the moment.

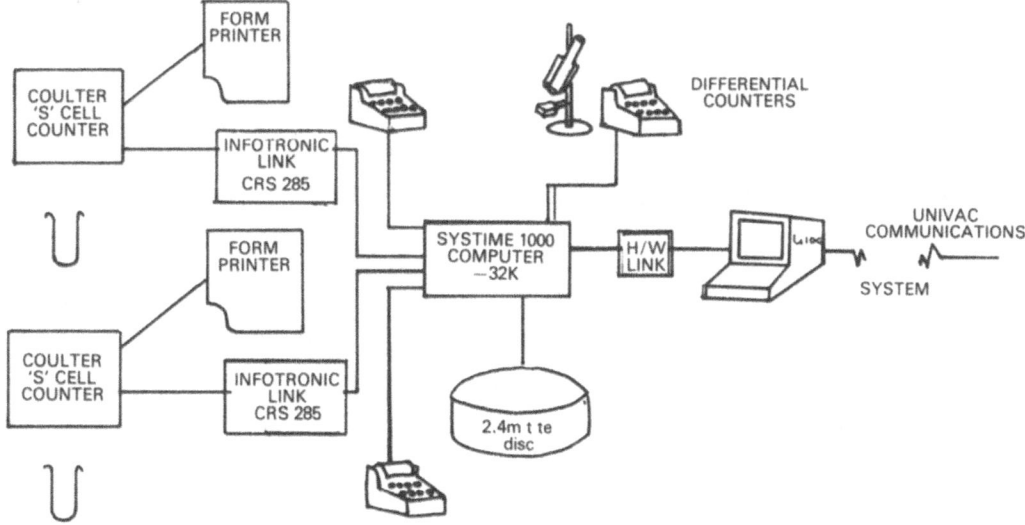

The haematology and blood transfusion link to the main frame computer.

Summary of Computerised Pathology System

1. Request via Ward Terminal
2. Printing of Request and Labels in Collection Schedule
3. Specimen Receipt Log-in
4. Printing of Laboratory Worksheets
5. On-line Capture of Results by Mini-Computers from:
    SMA Plus, Autoanalysers (x2), Coulter Counters (x2), Differential
    Counters (x6)
6. Approval of Results via VDU
7. Result Availability on Ward VDU's
8. Progress Queries on Ward VDU's
9. Cumulative and Individual Report Printouts

This would be a typical sequence of events. A request for blood would come via
a ward terminal. This is a particular difficulty for us because we shall not have
a houseman coming in with a blood specimen. He will sit somewhere away from the
laboratory, flash out a few things on the keyboard, and we get the bit of paper
at the other end. We then log the specimens in, print laboratory worksheets,
and we feel that in blood transfusion this will be particularly important. We
shall need worksheets in the laboratory.

The blood group serology and transfusion is in the same system. This merely
depicts the automatic equipment having a local storage computer before it is sent
off to the main frame system in another part of the hospital, and the results
becoming available on the VDUs.

Results are approved by VDU. Once we put it into the system it is available
all over the hospital. The doctor puts in his code, and no matter where he is,
he can find out the state of the crossmatch and whether his blood is ready, or not.
And so on.

We would be on-line through the local computer for blood transfusion work, and it
is through here we would hope to interface with Brentwood. But that would be for
our computer department to decide.

I have put the next illustration in not because it is anything special, but it is
perhaps topical since it is a modification of those gadgets that are used in
petrol stations. This local handset is a very good substitute for a very much
more expensive VDU. It is important, always, whenever staff are putting
information into a computer, that they get a hard copy locally to know what
they have done. We insist on this all the way through the system, and we would

certainly wish to have it if we go on-line to the blood transfusion centre.

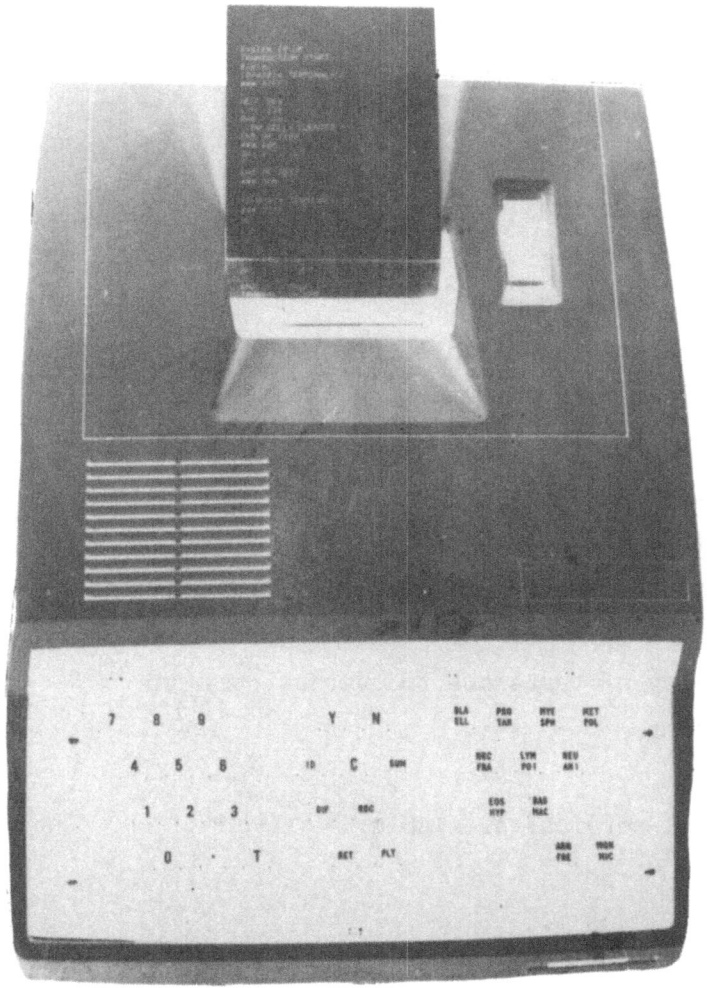

The next points show some of the advantages of our system.

Benefits to Doctors

1. Convenience

    a.   cumulative presentation.

    b.   progress of test can be ascertained.

    c.   requesting can be done on the wards.

    d.   results are obtainable on the wards immediately the technician has completed his activities.

    e.   pre-scheduling of tests may be done 'n' days hence.

2. Transit Time Improvement

    a.   automation in the laboratory.

    b.   postal elimination.

    c.   scheduling of specimen collection and laboratory work.

    d.   less interruption of work for answering queries.

Benefits to the Laboratories

1. Better Use of Technicians

    a. automated work sheet production

    b. online capture of test results from automated equipment and calibration control.

2. Better Use of Clerks/Collectors

    a. reduction in enquiries

    b. elimination of filing

    c. elimination of photocopying

    d. automated preparation of collection schedule.

Benefits to all Staff

1. Legibility and Completeness

    Omissions from forms have dropped from 7.5% to 0.65%

2. Efficient Specimen Collection

    No delay

    No overlooking of tests due to overdue reminder

3. Specimens Labelling

These are the pathology services available.

```
PICKLES AMELIA                        (CHOOSE ONE TEST CATEGORY)

  1 BLOOD CHEMISTRY                 15 SPUTUM CULTURE
  2 URINE CHEMISTRY
                                    17 POST-OPERATIVE WOUNDS
  4 BLOOD GROUP SEROLOGY            18 WOUND SWAB CULTURE
  5 HAEMATOLOGY                     19 OTHER SWAB CULTURE
                                    20 WOUND DRAINAGE
  7 IMMUNOLOGY                      21 H V S
  8 SCREEN FOR SYPHILIS (A R T)
  9 VIRUS STUDIES                   23 C S F  TESTS
 10 BLOOD CULTURE                   24 FAECES TESTS
 11 OTHER BLOOD TESTS              25 OTHER TESTS

 13 CLEAN M S U TESTS               88 DIALYSIS TESTS
 14 OTHER URINE TESTS            ▶ 1
```

Pictured below is an example of a request form generated by the system.

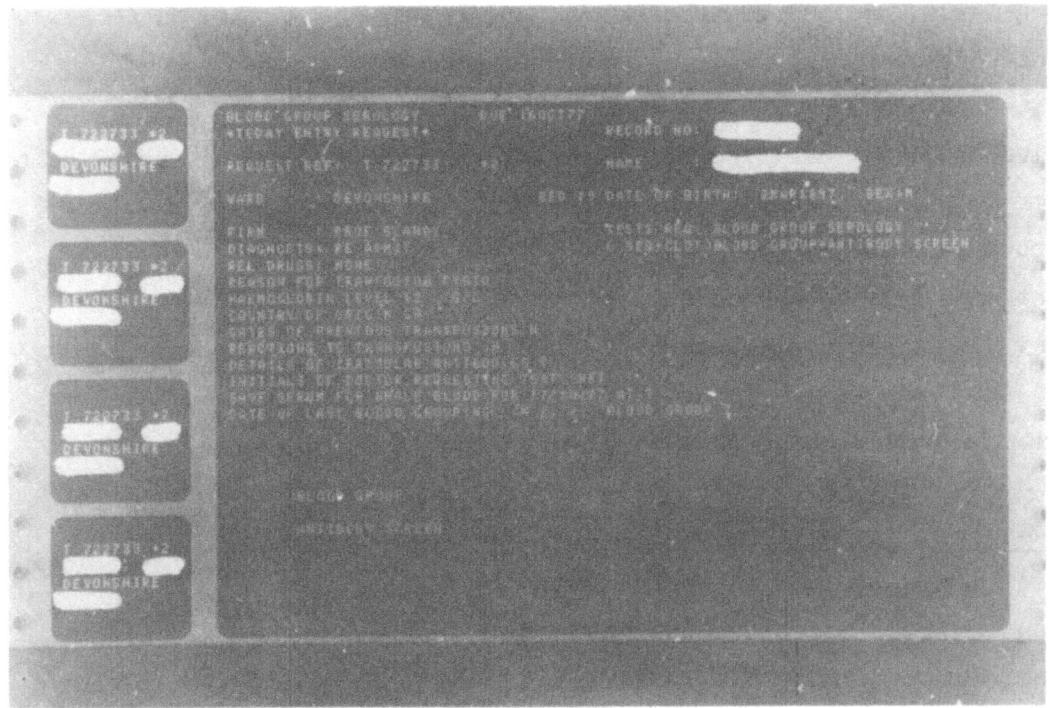

The detail does not much matter. Certain obligatory information must be
included as otherwise the request is not printed.

We collect all specimens for blood group serology unless it is an emergency
situation when the medical staff provide it. We get pre printed specimen
labels. I am sure that people will realise that this can be a dangerous part of
our system.

Recently we nearly had an accident because of this. It had nothing to do with
our on-line system, but whilst it is terribly convenient to have printed labels
it can be dangerous. The houseman took specimens of blood in the same ward. He
labelled the bottles with the official blood transfusion label. He then came down
to the laboratory, picked up the computer form with the printed labels, because
during the day they are printed in the laboratory and not in the computer centre,
tore off the labels and stuck them on to the wrong bottles. It was only because
the staff had remembered the names of the patients and had pulled the label back
that they noticed that he had really got the wrong patient in each instance.
When patients are anaesthetised there is no problem in getting blood in. The
implications are obvious. These labels carry a risk and we shall be re-examining
their safety.

Steps in Processing Laboratory Requests

1. Requesting from Ward Terminals + Specimen Collection.
2. Check-in of Specimen at Laboratory.
3. Print Logsheet.
4. Print Worksheets.
5. Derive Results - Assisted by Local Computers in Haematology and Biochemistry.
6. Enter Results - Directly from above Computers or Manually by V.D.U.
7. Approve Results.
8. Print and Distribute Reports.
9. Print Clinic Lists and Laboratory Records of Results.

Off-line result entries which could apply in blood transfusion

Offline Result Entry
Technician Records Results on Worksheet

Technician or Clerk Copies Results into VDU

Thereafter, Results May Be Viewed As "Unapproved", And Are Subsequently Validated.

Results Approval And Printing
Print "Approval Sheets" Showing Results Against Patient Details

Senior Staff Examine and Sign Approval Sheets

VDU Is Used To Signify Approval For Groups of Specimens

Subsequently, Reports Are Printed.

It is clear that at points within the system we are dealing with manual transcription and this carries an error rate. These are the sort of things we want to do away with by wanding with a light pen.

We also have a result approval and printing. This is the reporting end. Any result must be approved by the laboratory, by whoever is delegated to do it, before it is released. It is available on the VDUs immediately it is done in the laboratory. It is flagged as unapproved and anybody who takes action on that report must know that it has not been validated. We have an approval system which must be carried out, and the same thing would apply to blood issue.

I have shown these illustrations to give some insight into the system that we have in the hospital. We feel that we can fit in on-line to Brentwood with great advantage to the laboratory and to the patients.

There are several ways we can go about this. We can have a stand alone system

in the laboratory, purely for stock control, with a VDU, a light pen and a
printer, and one can just look up the stock control as one wishes. We would wish
to extend that further with an added facility - which is what we have provided
in the hospital - for inputs of patient details and subsequent printout for
distribution to the patient's notes. A record, a hard copy, must always be sent
to the patient's notes. Or, both could be rolled together, with an on-line
facility, allowing the clinician facility to use the ward VDU for looking up state
of progress of requests for blood, and when it is available how much has been
cross-matched and how much has been used.

Wanding out of blood from the laboratory to a particular patient can be done
locally, either by the patient being allocated a specific number with a check
digit by the computer system. We solidly believe in check digits. Or, possibly,
a local production of the bar code for attaching to the request form and specimen,
whereby a form generated in the laboratory is sent to the ward with patient's
record number with bar code attached. These are the difficult areas. The bar
code will identify the patient positively within certain limits, but a master
index is needed to make the system work. It has the disadvantage that
someone has to attach the bar codes to the form and we do not feel that this
will be a particularly attractive way to ensure positive patient identification.

These systems suffer from transcription error. Ideally we feel that patients will
need to be issued with a bar code version of their medical record number on
admission. I wonder whether this is realistic, and the administrators will
certainly query the cost. It would seem to be impossible to apply it solely
to the patients needing transfusion. That could be done in a proportion of cases,
but not in all. It could only be done by issuing codes to all admissions. To
this end, the way in for the hospital, is, I am sure, to have a facility locally
for producing a bar code identification of the patient. It is a computing problem
to line up the patient identification with any units of blood that are assigned
to that particular patient.

We feel that if generated in the laboratory, it would be a simpler business to get
the bar code on to the wrist band, and we should certainly be able to attach it to
the form and the specimen from the patient. That is the way we are thinking at
the moment. Reading of the wrist band in the ward, which would be the next stage
before it goes up on the hook, could be done either by an on-line system - there
are VDUs in all the wards so that would be quite easy for us. Alternatively it
could be done on a local tape storage and taken to the computer later on.
However, this would not be entirely satisfactory, and an on-system is needed for

the clinical staff to be certain that they have the right unit for the right
patient.

At the moment the hospital laboratories have a bar coding system on another piece
of apparatus just introduced into the hospital, a differential classifier. This
identifies patients by their record number, having been put on in the laboratory,
and by interfacing with our computer to the master index the patient and the
number are aligned. Any errors are picked up and we know when a mistake has been
made. I was interested to hear Dr Brodheim talk about locally producing bar
codes. I am sure we could devise other systems but I feel that this has probably
to be controlled from the laboratory. Otherwise forms will be arriving without
codes, or codes without forms, and we shall get into a thorough mess.

Any blood not used should, on return to the laboratory, be wanded back into the
system and flagged as returned blood. This would be for the blood transfusion
centre's information. Storage facilities in most wards are far from ideal, and
returned blood would have to be marked as such. As ever this would need
discipline, but the blood transfusion laboratory should know from the VDU screen,
what has been used and what is left, and it would be the laboratory's problem to
reclaim that blood. Blood which is time expired could be automatically removed
from the file, but we should not get this very often because stock control from
the centre should remove the need.

We do hope with the involvement of our computer department, and the active
participation of Brentwood to attempt to work out a system of patient recording
and identification of transfusion using bar code systems. In the first instance,
we would have a simulation exercise in the hospital to try to get our lines of
communication right before actually involving the transfusion centre. This is a
study that I hope will be put in hand fairly soon. We might perhaps confine it
to the operating theatre or the intensive care unit, not using a bar code, but
using a marker, so that we - through the management sciences staff - could get a
system before introducing a pilot study actually using the bar code.

Those are a few of our current thoughts. We have not had a lot of time to devote
to it, but we feel that any system that could add to patient safety must be
considered. Bar coded information with light wanding, doing away with manual
transcription, should be actively pursued, and particlarly for blood transfusion.

GENERAL DISCUSSION

Chairman: Dr W J Jenkins

Dr IBBOTSON: Might I start with a fairly vexed area - the quality control of printing of the Codabar labels. Has Dr Brodheim any experience of this? Do they check labels as they come into the centre or do they rely on the quality control of their printers?

Dr BRODHEIM: We do check the labels when they come into the centre. I am not happy with the quality control, either by the printers or in the centre. In my opinion we currently rely far too much on visual checking, which is error prone and which does not detect unreadable bar codes. I believe it would be much preferable to have checking done by reading immediately after printing. When we go to our in-centre printing of unit number labels we shall be attaching a laser device to the printer to read the labels immediately after printing and to verify that the numbers are both correct and readable.

Dr IBBOTSON: Has poor quality and unreadable labels been much of a problem?

Dr BRODHEIM: Not as much recently as at the beginning. For a year we were plagued by this problem. We had to go back and - with the collaboration of the manufacturer - revamp the whole quality control procedure until we reached the point we are at now where the quality is much better, and overall satisfactory. But - as Dr Bird pointed out - not without an occasional foul up.

Dr JENKINS: Would Dr Brodheim give us an idea of the availability of these printers. Obviously his centre will have to try them out, but if everything is successful will they be easily available, and how expensive?

Dr BRODHEIM: No. The preliminary pricing is that the printer itself will cost somewhere between $6,000 to $10,000. The label verification system, necessary in my opinion - but others may disagree, - will probably add an extra $4,000 to the

cost, which, with verification, means a total of $10,000 to $14,000. In my
opinion, for it to run properly it requires to be driven by the same mini-computer
that is controlling the other aspects of the label usage.

Dr JENKINS: In Dr Brodheim's case, this machine would be installed in a very
large centre, and its capability is much greater than that of a single centre in
the UK.

Dr BRODHEIM: The prototype device is to be installed in the Long Island
Center of the New York Blood Program which has been chosen for the experimental
work because it is fairly typical in size of most blood centres - approx 100,000
units collected per year. The capacity of the printer is several times as large
as is required.

Dr JENKINS: So it might be possible to group centres.

Dr BRODHEIM: Yes, and it would also be highly advisable to do so for many
reasons.

Dr NAPIER: We seem to have heard about a very secure system which seems to
begin with grouping and then proceed on to the issue of blood. Where we are still
vulnerable seems to be in ensuring that every constituent part of a donation is
correctly labelled.   That is an area that certainly concerns us - to ensure that
the bag, the testing samples and the record card all have exactly the same label.
I am wondering what experience there is of systems to cover weaknesses in this
area.

Dr BRODHEIM: Dr Napier is correct in that that is a matter of concern. What is
to be done about it is connected with the protocol for sticking unit numbers on to
the various items. In the US, most centres only apply unit numbers after the
donor has been screened and is accepted as a donor, which means that of necessity
they are applied at the collection site. It is possible to verify that they are
all the same and we have devised - on paper - a protocol for doing so. The
problem is that in order to implement the protocol, a portable device is needed

80

for doing it. I am not sure that a microprocessor would survive transport
to collection sites given our transport conditions in the US. We are hoping
for hand-held devices which would be the size of personal computers. These would
have memory, would be programmable to a limited extent, and could use the light
pen attachment. Such a device would also be used, or would be intended to be
used,for bedside verification of matching the patient identification - I should
say proposed patient identification - with the blood unit number. We are seeking
to have such a prototype device made. In my opinion, the technology exists for
doing this today, and I am hopeful that within one to two years, assuming we can
get the funding, such a device can be made and tested. In my opinion, such a
device is needed to make this practical. I do not believe that microprocessors
could practicably be carried around and set up at collection sites.

Dr CASH: I am pleased to hear that. We have difficulty in keeping our robust
donor beds intact and I am sure that existing microprocessor units would not
last more than a few sessions.

Dr BIRD: First, the format of the eye-readable portion of the labels. At
present this is in what I might call an 'ordinary' format. At a recent meeting
held in Geneva under the auspices of the ISBT it was reported that the Finns,
and the Swedes,have decided not to use the bar coding system but to go in for a
numerical system called OCR-B. It occurred to the meeting that this problem could
be easily solved if the eye-readable portion of the labels was actually in the
OCR-B format. Those who read these labels by eye can readily read what is written
in this format, and on an international level it keeps the Finns and the Swedes
happy.

Dr BRODHEIM: Recalling the very early label design, the eye-readable numbers
were in a very peculiar format. That is because they were in OCR-A which was
found to be totally unsatisfactory. OCR-B is quite acceptable, and it is a very
acceptable font to the eye. Theoretically what Dr Bird says can be done, and
should probably be done for practical purposes. For example, on sample tubes,
the system developed in Finland would be applicable.

I want to add a word of warning. OCR-B has a very high substitution error rate
compared to Codabar and consequently requires not one, but probably double the

check digits. In my opinion that eliminates much of the supposed advantage of OCR-B in that it clutters an already long number with two more digits, the eye cannot readily read bar code even if it feels like it, and can easily ignore it, but it cannot ignore extra printed numbers which are the same size and have the same appearance as the others.

Secondly, OCR, unlike Codabar, is very positional sensitive. We can stick two Codabar bar codes next to each other and read across them. We cannot do that with OCR. The pen has to be removed after every message and placed down again.

Thirdly, for OCR to read with any kind of reliability, control characters have to be put at both ends of the message.

It is my personal opinion that by the time all this is done it is not all that practical. I would agree that on general principle, since we have to print the eye-readable data anyway we might as well print it in the OCR-B format.

There is a fourth disadvantage, and I think it is a serious one. OCR has been standarised on 0.108 inches in height. When we tried it in the US, many blood bankers claimed that they could not read those numbers. Very often when they have a tight refrigerator they have to read these numbers from a considerable distance, and they were having problems reading numerals in OCR height.

OCR-B has limited application. For labels to go on sample tubes, fine, but to try to use it on the blood bag itself is - in my opinion - not viable.

Dr JENKINS: I would have thought that the transfer of blood between Scandinavia and the other Western countries, particularly the UK, is so limited as not to justify the use of OCR.

Dr BIRD: I raised this issue with my tongue in my cheek. Likewise the next issue, the question of colour coding. Is this really necessary? Historically there have been previous attempts at an international level which failed for obvious reasons. There are all manner of colours extant in various parts of the world and it became abundantly obvious that if a uniform colour coding system was to apply for the whole world this would run into all sorts of problems, not only on reaching agreement. Furthermore the stronger-minded people who might triumph in getting acceptance for a particular system might put the weaker-minded people in various parts of the world in much trouble by causing them to have to change the colour of their blood group labels.

A number of people who had given the matter some thought decided that these colours were not really necessary, and have given them up without experiencing any problems at all.

What are the views of the Meeting? We know that our own "users" here in the UK like colours and would like them to stay.

Dr GUNSON: We have discussed the use of plain labels at one meeting of the Working Party. It was agreed that at this stage their use should be rejected for two reasons, one of which Dr Bird has given ie it is well established practice in the UK to have colour coding for blood group labels. Secondly it was considered that as we were proposing many changes to the format of the labels, to abolish colour coding at the same time would be unacceptable.

Dr ROGERS (Tooting): Why do people want to take the colours off? There has been a lot of talk about standardisation and every system being the same, but how much blood is taken abroad from one country to another where the colours are different? Where blood is shipped abroad it is usually for a very specific purpose and they can take what precautions they feel are necessary in the country of reception.

Dr BRODHEIM: The only time the Committee for Commonality did not reach consensus but had to make an adoption by majority vote was on this very peripheral - to the Committee - issue of colour. We agreed on every highly technical aspect of everything, but could not agree on the rather emotional issue of colour.

Let me explain what I think motivated the majority to vote to remove colour for a period of time in the US. That is the fact that even within the US we were not consistent in colour. Different blood centres were using different colours for the same blood type. The feeling was that all dangers being weighed, the danger of that exceeded any transitory danger of removing colour. The vote was to eliminate colour for a period of at least two years - long enough for memory to die away - and only reinstitute it after an international agreement on the uniformity of colour that should include the colour coding of antisera.

That was the US recommendation, but it was by majority vote, with some people very passionately dissenting.

Dr BIRD: We have all been discussing the quality of Codabar printing, but how consistently do the light pens work? I have been around and I have seen them working extraordinarily well in the various transfusion centres, but complaints have been heard from here and there that they sometimes do not work too well. Does anyone have any knowledge of how consistent or accurate these light pens are, or whether there is a lot we have to learn as to how we have to use them?

Dr BRODHEIM: Light pens give extremely good read rates once they are properly calibrated. In theory all light pens shipped are pre-calibrated, but that is only in theory. We have found that we had to recalibrate two-thirds of the light pens we received. Our suppliers have finally consented to put a calibration pattern on the inside cover of the light pen so that we no longer have to do that ourselves.

My experience is that they are good, and they are consistently good, but they must be properly threshholded. If they are not properly threshholded all sorts of weird effects will be seen.

Dr CASH: How often is it necessary to recalibrate? Are there problems of drift with age?

Dr BRODHEIM: We have only had to recalibrate one pen after approximately one year of use and we have not instituted a systematic programme for doing this. But, prudence would dictate that once a year would be an advisable interval to recalibrate.

Dr CASH: How did you know when you had to recalibrate?

Dr BRODHEIM: We started to get a very poor read rate.

Dr BIRD: I have also heard that there is a knack in using light pens and that it takes time to acquire it. I would not condemn them without proper trial.

Dr BRODHEIM: True. But the knack is acquired rather fast. We have a light pen read programme which is literally a practise programme and tells the person when he has read it and when not. About twenty minutes practise is all that is required. However, a word of caution here. Different light pens have different characteristics. Some pens are much more difficult to use than others in that they are much more critical as to the angle at which they can be held, and so on. There is a substantial difference there. The easier ones require some training, but rather little.

Dr BIRD: I believe that speed is important and that it should not be done too slowly or too fast, and that the speed must be uniform.

Dr BRODHEIM: There is quite a dynamic range allowed. It will take something like a 5:1 or 6:1 range in speed. The trouble with most people not used to using a light pen is that they read much too slowly. There is a minimum. People are much more likely to get below the minimum speed than to exceed the maximum, and it is pretty hard to exceed the maximum speed. Most people cannot move their hands that quickly.

Dr BIRD: I like the rather satisfying ping that it makes when it gets it right and I feel sorry that it is not rigged to blow a raspberry if it gets it wrong.

Dr M FISHER (Oxford): We have only been using bar code labels with a GROUPAMATIC and we are about to use them on the blood packs with a light pen. Does handling, wetting of the packs, smearing of the labels, etc, affect readability, and what is the policy when this happens?

Dr BRODHEIM: Readability depends very much on whose labels are being used. I believe that Oxford is using Computype labels. They stand up to almost any kind of environmental conditions because they are on photographic film which is virtually immune to any of the normal damaging effects. Labels printed on paper stock are much more sensitive. Unless properly treated they will smear. When they are left in water the bar codes tend to run, which can make them unreadable. Some paper stock also scratches when a light pen is moved over it. It depends very much on the labels, on what kind of stock and what treatment is applied to the stock.

If one is unable to read, an unreadable label code can be scanned on the control sheet. At that point the computer will prompt the user to key the number in and verify it. In other words, every keying operation is required to be done twice. Not that that guarantees that one will not make the same mistake twice, but it is a little better.

Dr WAGSTAFF: To take that one step further. If the number is to be keyed in, then presumably the program must be so arranged that the group cannot be keyed in. The group must be fed in by light pen or someone would get round the label validation part. Is that right?

Dr BRODHEIM: As a matter of fact it is wrong. Probably it should be that way, but it is not that way. The way we have it set up now is that both the unit number and the blood type have to be keyed in. Dr Wagstaff is probably right in the sense that we should have broken it up and scanned the blood type in anyway, but we did not do so.

Dr JENKINS: It has been suggested that most of the information should be removed from the existing blood pack label but distributed in another form, and that people should be referred to a booklet for example. The Working Party would like to see that happen in the UK because it will leave room on the label to copy the American system. For the moment we have produced a compromise label to allow us to get off the ground.

Are there any feelings either way on removing that information from the labels?

Dr IBBOTSON: A corollary question to that. Where will the compatibility label be stuck? Is it to be tied on? If it is stuck on to the front then this information will be included and the donation number and blood group will need to be included. It is not a new question.

86

Dr JENKINS: It is very much in the hands of the individual hospitals. We must extend our influence into the hospitals when we design a new label with bar coding. In our region we ask the hospitals to stick such labels on to a tie-on label because blood is cross-matched so many times, and it might be very dangerous to have the label actually stuck on the bag. It varies enormously at the moment and there is a lot of tidying up to be done.

Dr IBBOTSON: It varies from hospital to hospital. Some people have mixed feelings about tie-on labels.

Lt Col THOMAS: I feel strongly, and have for a long time, about all the 'verbiage' to be found on a blood pack. I am sure it is there for exactly the same reason as the young casualty officer X-rays every sprained ankle that comes in. It is purely there as a 'cover'. The more writing there is on a pack, the less chance there is that the people who should read it will read it. I do not believe that the average transfusion technician needs to read it, because whether he be in a transfusion centre or in a hospital blood bank, he should be well enough versed by doing it often enough. What is written there should really be aimed at the people on the ward. It is the experience of those of us who have worked mainly in the clinical situation that the major problems of incompatible transfusion etc come from the people failing to read even such basics as the patient's name. The majority of incompatible transfusions are clearly labelled with the correct patient's name but are given to the wrong patient in spite of this.

A whole lot of small print jargon will not be read, especially in the emergency situation when the major danger arises.

One clear warning should be on the bag, roughly as Dr Brodheim suggested, written in red 'Are you giving this to the right patient?' That is really what we want to get across. Not something long and involved about the content, or how much ACD there is and make sure it is not wet, and wipe its bottom, and so forth. It is a load of garbage and it could well go off.

Can I ask where the Army blood supply depot fits into centre ID codes. We have no DHSS number.

Dr JENKINS: You can have one!

Lt Col THOMAS: I asked quite seriously. We already have laser readers and
it would be very nice to go back and to say that we want to fit in with the NBTS.
But one of the things we would need to say is that because a lot of our blood
goes out into the NHS, we should have a number so that our identification number
tied to our donor number makes a once-only number.

Dr JENKINS: I suggest that Colonel Thomas writes to Dr Gunson, who is Secretary
of the Working Party.

We are trying to persuade other regional centres to ship blood through the appropriate
local centre. Would this be very difficult for the Army?

Lt Col THOMAS: Frequently I will get a call from a hospital saying that they have
tried such and such a centre, they have none and can we let them have it. For us
then to ship it to wherever the regional centre is to ship to that hospital --
fair enough, but it is adding time especially with frozen blood. We ship frozen
blood to hospitals in at least three regions, and frozen blood has a shelf life
of twelve hours. If we have to ship it from us to the regional centre to the
hospital, that will probably waste six hours of the shelf life of that blood, and
when four units are being shipped for a child thalassaemic, it might be all the
difference between getting the blood into the patient inside its expiry time and
not getting it in.

Dr JENKINS: The problem arises when the patient gets some NBTS blood and some
army blood and then gets hepatitis. We are contacted, and we start tracing the
record not knowing that this patient has had blood from Army supply, and we
finally blame some donor of our own for what the Army has done. This is where
the confusion arises after the event.

Lt Col THOMAS: The other point is that we run a roll over system - no other
transfusion service runs one. Our lower user rate hospitals get issued with
blood which is withdrawn at the end of the week which moves on to a higher user
rate hospital, and then moves on in the third week to the high user NHS hospitals.
We do something which the NHS does not do. Because we have a much tighter
disciplinary control over our laboratories - in the strictest meaning of the

sense of the word 'disciplinary', we are much more confident that our blood is looked after the way we want it and is shipped the way we want it. So we are willing to receive blood back and to reissue it, which is not done in the NBTS.

Dr JENKINS: If the Army Blood Supply Depot would like a number it had best ask Dr Gunson who is at present allocating numbers.

Lt Col THOMAS: It is just that I think it would tidy things up neatly.

Dr JENKINS: Could we now discuss how we would introduce the simplified blood pack label?

Dr CASH: I would have thought that there would have to be two phases. One would be the provision of a label that could be used in Centres equipped with or without Codabar facilities. Such labels should contain the same basic information as those in current use. This approach would meet the urgent needs of some Centres. Phase two might be introduced after detailed reconsideration as to what information really needs to appear on a blood bag label. I would have thought that, aside from getting agreement of representatives of the Blood Transfusion Service, it would be essential to consult and obtain the agreement of the Government regulatory bodies. Simplification of the labels may make sense but it will probably have legal consequences.

Dr JENKINS: I would have thought that the first label is at least a year off and that we could stall its introduction so that all centres start together.

Dr CASH: I think it is important not to confuse the issue. As I understand it a modified label is one which contains all the information that is currently present. It has been redesigned in order to suit those wishing to use Codabar, but at no detriment to those who will not. The simplified label, as I understand it, is one which might be designed in the future, with the specific purpose of reducing the amount of detailed information. Such an exercise will take some time.

Dr JENKINS: But the modified label would be used in the meantime.

Dr GUNSON: To follow on Dr Cash's point on the ACD formula, is it necessary to give the recipe on the pack when one could refer to a Pharmacopoeia where the recipe is stated?

Dr CASH: Although I support such a move, I think we ought to bear in mind that although the formula for ACD may be standard, the volume of anticoagulant may not be identical from different manufacturers. This may interest the regulatory authorities and perhaps the plasma fractionators.

A W BARRELL (Travenol): We can start discussions with the necessary regulatory bodies once we know that there is agreement amongst those working in the transfusion service that the label should be modified and that that information can come off.

Dr JENKINS: I assume that our Working Party will put this to the RTD's as soon as possible to try to get a decision from the RTDs.

The FDA is held in high esteem in the UK. As I understand it, the FDA has agreed to this.

Dr BRODHEIM: No. The FDA has not. However, the problem is not as bad as it seems. The recipe for CPD must appear on the label but only until it is filled. What we do is to put it on the part that is later covered by the blood type label, so that it takes no space at all.

Dr CLEGHORN (Edgware):   All these regulatory bodies are allowing these bags to
go out grossly mislabelled in any event because they state when they are empty
that they contain human blood!

Mrs WILD: I believe I am right in saying that the Medicines Act specifies that
if the title of the product is quoted with its BP reference it is not necessary
to give the components. If it quoted as 'anti-coagulant BP' the formulation can
be obtained by direct reference to the Pharmacopoeia.

Lt Col THOMAS: I still have a point to take up with Dr Cash.I do not believe
at the present moment that what is written is there because of any law that says
that it has to be there. We have put it there because we wish to cover ourselves
against any danger that may happen. We can say that if such and such was not done
it should have been done because it was written on the pack. I do not believe it
is beyond the wit of the DHSS to issue a circular. It could then be printed on
the pack; 'Compliance must be with Hospital Circular .....' which would list this
information plus a lot more. One needs a degree of understanding before one can
interpret what is at present written on the pack. Therefore, what is there is
not in itself complete. It needs more explanation. For example: 'transfusion
set must have a filter.' Does that mean a piece of filter paper? It is only
people with a certain amount of education who will know the sort of filter that
we are talking about and that it has to be in line. 'Contents must not be used if
there is visible evidence of deterioration.' People have to be taught what visible
evidence of deterioration is. They have to look for a mauve line.

I believe that what is important, what causes the problem 99 times out of 100, is
an administrative clerical error in the transfusion. That is why it is important
to have written in huge letters: 'Check that this is the right patient.' The
rest of it can be 'please ensure that this complies with hospital circular No ...'
I do not think the present wording covers everything, and yet I do think it is
verbose; therefore, falling between two stools.

Dr CASH: Whilst I have considerable sympathy, and feel able to support most of Lt Col Thomas' remarks, I must point out that if change is required it will have to be cleared by the appropriate regulatory bodies. It will not, in my view, be acceptable to make a unilateral change in the contents of a label and simply refer the clinician to a hospital Circular. For good or evil, those days have gone.

It is intersting that many labels on the containers of fractionated blood products are very sparse, but it is my impression that the regulatory authorities insist that each vial delivered to the bed-side is in a box which contains a leaflet giving much detailed information. We may have something to learn from this approach. Nonetheless I would again advise caution with regard to change, particularly at the present time, as the question of legal liability for product defects is currently under scrutiny and part of this debate is about the informed consent of patients and the duty of the manufacturer to see the prescribing doctor is appropriately informed.

Lt Col THOMAS: There is definitely a problem of what is informed consent. If the patient is consenting to blood transfusion exactly to what is he consenting? Consent is not valid unless it is informed consent and exactly how many patients give informed consent to a blood transfusion?

I should like to take up one point about these labels. In the British Pharmacopoeia it states that all Group O blood should state on the label whether or not it is high-titer, whether it has been tested for haemolysins. I noticed that the stick-on labels do not mention that 'O' blood has been so tested, and that is a pharmacopoeial requirement.

Dr JENKINS: We do use such labels, but they form another series which is not bearing a bar code.

Lt Col THOMAS: But the British Pharmacopoeia states that Group O blood must state that it has been tested for haemolysins, and it is either positive or negative for haemolysins. These labels do not carry that requirement which is a requirement of the BP at the present time.

Dr JENKINS: It is also necessary to test for hepatitis, for syphilis, and so on, but we do not put all that on the labels.

Lt Col THOMAS: We have it on ours. All the Army labels say: Group; negative for VD reagin test; negative when tested for hepatitis; HBsAg. And the 'O' labels have negative for haemolysins. That is actually printed on every label.

Dr CASH: That is an interesting point, but not quite appropriate to our original topic. We were discussing the removal of existing information, whereas you are asking questions about the placing of additional information on blood bags. I suspect that regulatory authorities are less interested in the latter than the former. Nonetheless the points you have raised may well be relevant in the context of product liability and may, therefore, need to be considered in the design of a new blood bag label.

Dr JENKINS: We test all units for haemolysins, and if there is no label on it implies that there are no haemolysins present. But we certainly put a label on where there are, in the same way as we put on a bio-hazard label if a unit is hepatitis positive.

Dr BIRD: It was only last Friday that I said to another gathering that I feared that soon we shall have so many labels that we shall not be able to see the blood at all.

Dr NAPIER: Putting the instructions on the bag might lead people to suppose that they were the only necessary instructions, whereas many hospital blood banks would regard their own standing orders for transfusion as being more explicit and more comprehensive. I do not think that these fulfil everybody's requirements in that respect, and that is an argument for not putting any instructions on the bag, apart, perhaps, from specific cautions about the need for identification of the recipient. The vagueness of instructions about use of a filter (ie what sort of filter) and the vagueness of instructions regarding identifying the recipient and the need for a cross-match are really not desirable. Reference to standard recommendations would be a much better alternative.

Dr JENKINS: Do I get you right, Dr Cash, that you are quoting the law?

Dr CASH: I am not a lawyer, nor do I know the law! I am, however, aware of the increasing activities of regulatory authorities in many countries, and would imagine that companies will not change existing blood bag labels without the formal approval of the appropriate authority in the UK.

Dr JENKINS: It is not the intention of our Working Party, or of the RTDs, and I'm sure its beyond the intention of Travenol, to make any of these changes without going through the whole procedure of obtaining authority to do so.

Mrs WILD: Products other than transfusion products which are infused do not carry all kinds of warnings. They carry some printed on the pack itself. But there is a requirement to include certain information in each carton of product that is shipped.

For straight IV fluids - dextrose, saline etc we do not give specific directions for use of the solution. We use a statement referring back to a data sheet and we refer to directions for use.

The directions for use refer to the use of the container and not to the actual use of the product.

Dr CASH: That is quite right, but we may have to be careful that information on blood bag labels which becomes formulised by regulatory authorities can be backed up by specifications which are acceptable and achievable. For instance, I would imagine that we will readily agree on a label entitled, 'Platelet Concentrate'. However, I believe a regulatory authority will require a specification and an acceptable programme of quality control which seeks to confirm that the specification is being met. Such developments have considerable financial implications to the Transfusion Service.

Dr IBBOTSON: We have departed somewhat from the Commonality Commission in that they are printing on their product labels some critical bits on storage conditions. We have been shown 'use an on-line filter for platelets'. They are

94

printing storage temperatures. We jumped the gun somewhat in Birmingham in that we had to have the product labels·printed before they were agreed in the Working Party. We followed the American Code of Practice in this - and it is a little bit larger than the version finally accepted by the Working Party.

Is there an argument for putting on the critical bits regarding storage conditions?

Dr CASH: At the present time I would not be in favour of this, partly because there is no good agreement on many of these details: they remain somewhat controversial.

Dr GUNSON: That is correct, particularly in the case of platelet concentrates where one must advise a particular storage temperature which may be in dispute but in general alteration in the size of the labels must wait until we have agreement on the redesigned pack label for the future. If the product labels are made larger now they will cover up some of the writing on the front face of the pack. The Working Party considered this aspect as one for future development.

Dr CASH: I would like to ask Dr Brodheim what he does with his Codabar arrangements when for instance he issues a platelet concentrate or cryoprecipitate in a single bag that is derived from 6 or 12 donations?

Dr BRODHEIM: We have a product code for what we call multiple donor units. If, say, twelve units of platelets are pooled then that is basically destroying twelve products and creating a new product. In other words, the twelve products that have gone into the pooled units have disappeared giving a new unit with a new reference number. The blood centre will maintain the association, so if a hepatitis traceback needs to be done, the record exists.

What happens is that those twelve products are disposed of and a new uniquely numbered product has been created in their place.

Dr CASH: We use an increasing number of our donations, for reagents - what type of label would be used for this type of donation?

Dr GUNSON: Not specifically for laboratory use. There will be a label available which states 'not for transfusion' which has space available for giving the reason. Such a label could be used for a laboratory reagent in the present system.

Lt Col THOMAS: How much extra is this to cost? Do Travenol foresee that this will put up the cost of the packs, and what is the estimated cost of the Codabar labels to go on to the packs? I know the cost of the individual sets of numbers, but what will the actual 'A' positive and 'B' positive labels be costing over and above what we now pay?

Dr GUNSON: The group labels which I have described have competitive prices with the labels used previously in the Oxford Region.

Lt Col THOMAS: And the cost of the packs? Will it become more expensive to have this put on the packs as far as Travenol are concerned, and will Travenol put out packs with our address and our particular unit designation on them in Codabar?

A W BARRELL (Travenol): Changing the label to accommodate Codabar will not change the cost of the pack. We are not anticipating any price increase in changing the label.

In terms of the eventual provision of labels we have agreed to support the initial supplies of stick-on labels. We have said that we shall look at the possibility of future supply, and we have to look at that in terms of the cost. We have not calculated costs to see how much that might entail.

Dr JENKINS: But it should be trivial because these labels are extremely simple. Other than the blood group labels they are very simple labels.

A W BARRELL (Travenol): Yes. I should like to think that if it is what is wanted we are able to accommodate that.

96

Dr JENKINS: My fear is that if we do not channel these standarised labels
through one source, over the course of a few years modifications will be made
by individual centres and we shall be back in a few years' time to a variety of
different wordings and different labels. It is only if we can get a central
source for these labels that they would only be modified by consensus - which
would be the Working Party. People would put up good reasons for changing the
wording and everybody would change together. This would be far more satisfactory.

Dr CASH: Whereas I would strongly support the principle of a central house -
surely this cannot be a single blood bag manufacturer?

A W BARRELL (Travenol): But it would not be. This would be a printer of stick-
on labels. We have no desire or intention to get into the printing business,
neither do we have any desire to become the distributors of labels. What we are
saying is that to assist the scheme to get started, and to continue if it is
desired that we should continue. We would support the provision of labels, but
those labels would come directly from the printer to the transfusion centre.
Otherwise, the logistical difficulty that can occur when lines of communication
are lengthened might make life difficult for everyone.

Lt Col THOMAS: Purely a look into the future: is there any way that the
'pigtails' - so my technicians call the pack tube which at the present moment
has the once only numbers - could carry a Codabar? In clinical practice, if this
is to be taken into the hospital laboratory it might be very useful where there
are four or five transfusions set up to be able to zip up the bit that has been
put off and cut into a tube where those cells are being used to set up a
crossmatch, and to run that against the Codabar on the pack. I realise that
there are obviously problems because it is stretchable, and this sort of thing,
but is it something that is being looked at?

Dr BRODHEIM: It was looked at. We had gotten fairly far with our Symbol
Selection Task Force working with Travenol in the US and Travenol's conclusion
was that it could be done. Then we had a very interesting situation where our
labelling task force suddenly decided that they did not think it was necessary,
so the project was dropped. The recommendation was that when segments are used
they are invariably - and I am not stating a personal opinion I am merely giving
the recommendation - they are invariably placed within a test tube in any event.

The test tube could be properly identified, and they felt that it was necessary to put the machine readable code on the segments.

The technical opinion was that it could be done. Fenwal had indicated that they were willing to do it, and then our Committee dropped the requirement.

I can only report that the technical appraisal was that it could be done but it was not done.

Dr JENKINS: One of the problems is that that number can never be the same as the number awarded at the time of donation, so there would be two numbers to collate all the time.

Lt Col THOMAS: That number could be on the pack itself.

Dr BRODHEIM: That is harder to do. It is much harder to do because of the way the bags are manufactured. The segments are produced and then they are put on the pack. It would be very difficult.

However, a one-time collation of the unit number at the time it appeared at the hospital with the internal hospital number can be readily done.

A computer system in a hospital would mean that that correlation need be done only once, and thereafter it could be interchangeably worked with either number. So it is probably technically feasible to do so.

Lt Col THOMAS: The reason I ask is that it is connected with something we do that no other transfusion centre does. We group every pack by taking off a pigtail, and cell grouping that pigtail, and then that gets married. Before the packs go down into the blood bank they get married with the group that is done on the pilot tube. In other words, we group the specimen tube. We also take a pigtail from the pack and that is also grouped. Those two groups are married and if the two groups do not check --

Soldiers have a lovely habit of swapping round tubes and this sort of thing. It is not unknown for us to find that two blokes have swapped their tubes. When they come back into the centre we do not know this, so we always do this extra check of checking and making sure that the group that the person has been grouped with is the same as is in the pack. So it would be useful to us.

Dr JENKINS: This has been a most useful meeting for the members of the Working Party. May I thank all of you for attending and contributing to such a lively discussion. Especially, I thank Dr Brodheim, our principal speaker for coming all the way from New York to give us the benefit of his vast experience.

I am sure you would wish to express your thanks, through the chair, to all the speakers and, finally, to Travenol Laboratories for sponsoring this excellent meeting and for their generous hospitality.

Delegate list

Dr G W G Bird (Birmingham)
Dr E Brodheim (New York)
Dr J D Cash (National Director, Scotland)
Dr T E Cleghorn (Edgware)
Dr A Collins (Newcastle)
Dr J Darnborough (Cambridge)
Dr J England (Edgware)
Mr R G Fewell (The London Hospital)
Dr M Fisher (Oxford)
Dr H H Gunson (Oxford)
Dr R N Ibbotson (Birmingham)
Mrs S Jackson (Birmingham)
Dr W J Jenkins (Brentwood)
Dr R Lane (Lister Institute, Elstree)
Dr W J Lockyer (Bristol)
Dr W M McClelland (Belfast)
Dr J A F Napier (Cardiff)
Dr F M Roberts (Liverpool)
Dr H E Roberts (Sheffield)
Dr K L Rogers (Tooting)
Miss S Rosbotham (DHSS)
Dr D S Smith (Southampton)
Prof F Stratton (Manchester)
Lt Col M Thomas (Army BTC)
Dr W. Wagstaff (Sheffield)
Dr J Wilkinson (Dublin)
Mr G Williams (Brentwood)
Mr A W Barrell (Travenol)
Mrs A Wild (Travenol)

GPSR Compliance

*The European Union's (EU) General Product Safety Regulation (GPSR)
is a set of rules that requires consumer products to be safe and our
obligations to ensure this.*

*If you have any concerns about our products, you can contact us on
ProductSafety@springernature.com*

In case Publisher is established outside the EU, the EU authorized
representative is:

Springer Nature Customer Service Center GmbH
Europaplatz 3
69115 Heidelberg, Germany

Batch number: 09635764

Printed by Printforce, the Netherlands